PENGUIN CLASSICS  DELUXE EDITION

KAMA SUTRA

VATSYAYANA composed the *Kama Sutra* after careful study and consideration "while observing a celibate's life in full meditation." Very little else is known about him. His first name was perhaps Mallanaga and from his detailed descriptions of regional practices, we can surmise that he was from the Madyha Desha, the then cultural heartland of India. He lived nearly two thousand years ago and this work was the first of its kind anywhere in the world. Cited repeatedly in Indian literature, it became known outside that country just over a century ago and has been a byword for eroticism ever since.

ADITYA NARAYAN DHAIRYASHEEL HAKSAR is a well known translator of Sanskrit classics. He has also had a distinguished career as a diplomat, serving as Indian high commissioner to Kenya and the Seychelles, minister to the United States and ambassador to Portugal and Yugoslavia. His translations from the Sanskrit include *The Shattered Thigh and Other Plays*, *Tales of the Ten Princes*, *Hitopadesa*, *Simhasana Dvatrimsika*, *Subhashitavali,* and *Three Satires from Ancient Kashmir*, all published as Penguin Classics.

VATSYAYANA

Kama Sutra

A GUIDE TO THE ART OF PLEASURE

a new translation by
A. N. D. HAKSAR

PENGUIN BOOKS

PENGUIN BOOKS

Published by the Penguin Group
Penguin Group (USA) Inc., 375 Hudson Street, New York, New York 10014, U.S.A.
Penguin Group (Canada), 90 Eglinton Avenue East, Suite 700, Toronto,
Ontario, Canada M4P 2Y3 (a division of Pearson Penguin Canada Inc.)
Penguin Books Ltd, 80 Strand, London WC2R 0RL, England
Penguin Ireland, 25 St Stephen's Green, Dublin 2, Ireland (a division of Penguin Books Ltd)
Penguin Group (Australia), 250 Camberwell Road, Camberwell,
Victoria 3124, Australia (a division of Pearson Australia Group Pty Ltd)
Penguin Books India Pvt Ltd, 11 Community Centre, Panchsheel Park, New Delhi – 110 017, India
Penguin Group (NZ), 67 Apollo Drive, Rosedale, Auckland 0632,
New Zealand (a division of Pearson New Zealand Ltd)
Penguin Books (South Africa) (Pty) Ltd, 24 Sturdee Avenue,
Rosebank, Johannesburg 2196, South Africa

Penguin Books Ltd, Registered Offices:
80 Strand, London WC2R 0RL, England

First published in Great Britain by Penguin Classics 2011
Published in Penguin Books (USA) 2012

9th Printing

Translation copyright © A. N. D. Haksar, 2011
All rights reserved

LIBRARY OF CONGRESS CATALOGING IN PUBLICATION DATA
Vatsyayana.
[Kamasutra. English]
Kama sutra : a guide to the art of pleasure / by Vatsyayana ; a new
translation by A. N. D. Haskar.—Penguin classics deluxe ed.
p. cm.
Includes bibliographical references.
ISBN 978-0-14-310659-3
1. Love. 2. Sex. 3. Sex instruction. 4. Sex customs. 5. Vatsyayana. Kamasutra.
I. Haskar, A. N. D., 1933– II. Title.
HQ470.S3V31 2012
613.9'6—dc23   2011043102

Printed in the United States of America

P. M. S.

For
B.
with love

Contents

BOOK TWO: SEXUAL UNION

BOOK THREE: THE MAIDEN

CONTENTS

BOOK FOUR: THE WIFE

BOOK FIVE: WIVES OF OTHERS

BOOK SIX: THE COURTESAN

CONTENTS

BOOK SEVEN: ESOTERIC MATTERS

Introduction

The *Kama Sutra* was written in India nearly two thousand years ago. It is barely more than a hundred years since it became known outside the country of its origin. Interest in it seems ageless. In India it has been cited century after century in other works, as well as influencing literature and art. In the wider world its celebrity, or notoriety, remains unaffected by the information explosion on its principal subject in our times.

Present Perceptions

The title has 183 listings in the online catalogue of the US Library of Congress. These include several books with the original text and commentary in Sanskrit, the literary language of ancient India. Much more numerous are translations into English and other languages such as French, German, Italian and Russian, not to mention those of South Asia like Bengali, Hindi, Marathi and Telugu. There are also some scholarly studies of Indian history, literature and social life bearing on the work.

But more than half the titles in the Congressional list point to perspectives other than the academic. They range from

Complete Illustrated Kama Sutra to *Pocket Idiot's Guide to the Kama Sutra*, and from *Kitchen Kama Sutra: 50 ways to seduce each other outside the bedroom* to *Pop-up Kama Sutra: 6 paper-engineered variations*. The last entry is *Kama Sutra 52: A year's worth of best positions for passion and pleasure* published in 2009.

The work seems to have two popular reputations in the West, according to a recent commentator from the United Kingdom. One as an exotic compendium of positions for human copulation and the other 'as a repository of Oriental erotic wisdom, the Ur-text of a profoundly spiritual tradition'. Either way, he says, 'it has become a byword for sex itself.'[1] Also, one may add, a brand name for consumer marketing and advertisement, to go by the establishments and products which use its unpatented title.

This reputation also extends to modern India. Much of its vast population may yet be largely unaware of the work. But among many of its intellectual class the *Kama Sutra* 'is still held up as a proud example of that country's alternative tradition of sexual morality'.[2] A popular brand of condoms bears its name, as do many publications with colourful pictures in coffee-table and pocket-size editions. However, these are mostly bought by tourists, thinks an Indian psychoanalyst, scholar and novelist of the subject, and the locals 'don't read it any more; they only look at illustrations of the sexual positions'. What it is really about, he says, 'is the art of living – about finding a partner, maintaining power in marriage, committing adultery, living as or with a courtesan, using drugs – and also about positions in sexual intercourse. It has attained its classical status as the world's first comprehensive guide to erotic love because it is at the bottom about essential, unchangeable human attributes – lust, love, shyness, rejection, seduction, manipulation, that are also a part of human sexuality.'[3]

An Ancient Assessment

The repute of the *Kama Sutra* and its author in ancient India, and its position in the knowledge system of the time, is perhaps put most simply in another well-known and possibly not much later work. This is the *Panchatantra*, a popular collection of animal and human fables still in wide circulation. In the prologue of its text a king, anxious to have his children well educated, is told: 'Majesty, it is heard that grammar takes twelve years. Then come Manu and other works on Dharma, Chanakya and those on Artha, and Vatsyayana and others on Kama. Thus are the sciences of Dharma, Artha and Kama learnt. Then does knowledge develop.'[4] A subsequent tale in the same text (1.5) narrows the focus somewhat. In it a friend advises a lover to go to his beloved who is alone so that 'you may enjoy her in accordance with the methods prescribed by Vatsyayana.'[5]

Four things seem clear from these references in a book which was meant for instruction as well as entertainment. First, general education at the time was seen broadly to comprise three main branches of knowledge after reading, writing and grammar. Second, each of these had come to be identified with the work of one particular authority. Third, Kama was one of the three branches and the name associated with it was that of Vatsyayana. Finally, though Kama may have had a wider connotation inclusive of other pursuits, its principal concern was with sex.

The Three Ends

It is fitting first to consider the wider context. It conceptualized a trinity of worldly pursuits or ends of human life, summed up in the words Dharma, Artha and Kama. Each has multiple meanings but, very broadly, Dharma is virtue and righteous conduct, Artha is wealth, power and material well-being and Kama is desire for and sensual pleasure of all kinds. There were areas, such as marriage, where they overlapped. But each was seen as a basic motivator and goal of normal human action as a whole, and worthy as such of study and regulation. A well-rounded education presumed some familiarity with this triad (*trivarga*) of human objectives (*purushartha*), each with its due place in life. A fourth end, which made it a quartet (*chaturvarga*), was Moksha or salvation. But that was an other-worldly pursuit.

The three ends are spelt out briefly and clearly in the *Kama Sutra*'s Book One, Chapter 2. Their mutual relationship and comparative importance are also discussed, though with some ambivalence. While the pursuit of Dharma obviously took precedence over the other two, its benefits might accrue only in a future life. Artha, on the other hand, could be more important for people like kings and courtesans because of their worldly requirements. Kama was a basic need like food. The comparison was businesslike, but it could also be cynical, as shown by a later Sanskrit poet and author of a now lost commentary on the *Kama Sutra*:

> Talk of Dharma, taste for Kama,
> mind for Moksha, come about
> only when content and comfort

dawn in bellies taut with hunger:
for, when it is the time to eat,
and no money nor the means,
who thinks of Dharma, relishes Kama,
or looks to that which leads to Moksha?

and,

The ultimate fruit of wealth, they say,
can be a religious ceremony;
and that results, without dispute,
in merit which leads to paradise;
but paradise itself is simply
women in their sixteenth year.[6]

Be that as it may, the three ends formed an overall context for learning and conduct, within which Vatsyayana concentrated on a subject which was both sexual as well as social at the time. 'Its principal element', he says, 'is a delightful, creative feeling pervaded by sensual pleasure.'

The Author and the Times

The *Kama Sutra* names Vatsyayana as its author. He is also mentioned as such in a number of subsequent works. A fifth-century CE novel, *Vasavadatta* by Subandhu, names him Mallanaga. This, says a later commentator,[7] was his given name, Vatsyayana being the family name. The little that he has mentioned about himself is confined to his epilogue: how he composed the work after careful study and consideration of earlier material 'while observing a celibate's life in full meditation'. Nothing else is known about him. From his description of regional practices it is surmised that he may have been from the then cultural heartland of India, the Madhya Desha or central region; and may have lived in Pataliputra, its metropolis at the time, identified with a site near modern-day Patna.

The dating of the *Kama Sutra*, as with much ancient Indian chronology, is affected by the absence of conclusive data. Though there is no consensus on the subject, most scholars now place it in the third century CE.[8] This puts it after the other two works regarded as foundational texts of the then knowledge system: the *Manava Dharma Shastra* of Manu on the legal and social codes of conduct, and the *Artha Shastra* of Kautilya or Chanakya on economics and politics. With the latter it has stylistic similarities which some scholars think indicate that the *Artha Shastra* may have served as a model for Vatsyayana. He also knew other works like the *Atharva Veda* and the *Ayurveda*, which he mentioned in his text.

In historical terms this was a time between the dissolution of the Kushana and the rise of the Gupta empire in north India. Though a period of political transition, it was also marked by a continued flowering of knowledge and an expansion of trade and commerce, with consequent prosperity which provided the means and the leisure for aesthetic pursuits by the affluent. The *Kama Sutra* gives vivid accounts of these in its descriptions of the life of a gentleman and of professional courtesans who formed a class similar to the hetaeras of Greece and the geishas of Japan. This is the setting in which its examination of social and sexual behaviour is undertaken.

The Work's Genre and Contents

According to a recent study[9] the *Kama Sutra* is both descriptive and prescriptive, and comes in the category of *shastra*, the same as the works on Dharma and Artha already mentioned. 'The term has no exact parallel in English,' says Manu's latest translator. 'It may refer to a system, a tradition of expert knowledge in a particular field, that is, a science. It refers especially to the textualized form of that science i.e. an authoritative compendium of knowledge.'[10] Vatsyayana's work broadly fits this description. It is a treatise on Kama, in both the social and sexual aspects of human relationships. It quotes from earlier works, defines various dimensions of the subject and frames its descriptions and prescriptions in coldly clinical and generally dispassionate terms. A notable feature is its recurrent disclaimers. Their theme is that descriptions must not be considered as recommendations, and the latter must also take particular situations into account. This adds an intimate note to the otherwise impersonal, didactic approach.

Another seemingly personal touch comes through the verses which intersperse the text's prose. Their sources are not specified and some could well be of Vatsyayana's own composition. A refreshing counterpoint to the prose, which is framed in the *sutra* style of brief passages with compressed meaning in telegraphic language, the verses are in the more expansive *shloka* form well known through the great Indian epics. As in the *Artha Shastra*, they often provide a summation or make a point after the prose passages. A recent scholarly translation notes in its introduction that 'the prose, by and large, describes what people do; only in the verses does Vatsyayana explicitly suggest what people should do.'[11] Further, 'the voice of these verses is one of moderation and reason.' Also, it may be noted, of an occasional tongue-in-cheek scepticism which adds to the personal touch.

Described precisely in its first chapter, the *Kama Sutra*'s contents are spread over seven books and thirty-six chapters. In contrast to the image the work later acquired, only one of the seven books, the second, deals with the act of sex in its various aspects. The first book lays out the contextual background and describes the life of a gentleman, his social, romantic and other pursuits and the work of his aides. The third and the fourth discuss courtship, marriage and the role of the wife. The fifth book is concerned with extra-marital relations, in a mainly polygamous society, and with life in the harem. The sixth deals with the life and conduct of courtesans. The final book, which is more a collection of recipes than an analytical account, provides prescriptions for increasing attractiveness, stimulating passion, enhancing virility and exerting control over a partner. None of the books, it is interesting to note, appear to be exclusively for men; they also contain advice for maidens and wives, mistresses and courtesans: women are recognized as individuals.

The *Kama Sutra* was written during a period of economic growth with greater scope for elegant living, and of increased cultural activity, in a society which recognized the legitimacy of pleasure as a basic human pursuit, along with that of virtue and wealth. It expounded on the first, but also urged a balance with the other two, as is evident from the final verse of its epilogue. Its detailed expositions on the lifestyles of cultivated gentlemen and fashionable courtesans give some idea of the audience to which it was addressed. Later literary evidence would indicate that both used it as a guide for recreational and professional purposes. But it also dwells on other matters, specially of marital import: the aesthetic education of girls; the wooing of a prospective bride; the role of partners in matrimony, monogamous as well as polygamous; and also on romantic relationships outside marriage, apart from erotic techniques for the enhancement of sensual pleasure. It is thus a fairly comprehensive manual on loving and living, and deals both with contemporary issues and others which are timeless.

Influence on Later Literature

As already mentioned, Vatsyayana is cited by name in the fourth-century CE *Panchatantra*[12] and the *Kama Sutra* in the fifth-century novel by Subandhu. The language and the terminology of the work are thought to have been reflected in descriptions of the courtesan and the gentleman in Shudraka's fourth-century play *Mriccha-katika* (*The Little Clay Cart*); in amorous episodes in Kalidasa's fifth-century epic poems *Kumarasambhava* and *Raghuvamsha*; in the love lyrics of the eighth-century *Amarushatakam*; and in the ecstatic songs of Jayadeva's twelfth-century *Gitagovinda*. Though none of these famous works actually cite the *Kama Sutra* or its author, such references are found in later Sanskrit commentaries on some of them.[13] Citations also exist in other works, like the seventh-century epic poem *Shishupalavadha* of Magha and the eighth-century satire on courtesans *Kuttanimatam* of Damodaragupta.

Apart from its reflection in the subsequent poetical literature of Sanskrit, the *Kama Sutra* also inspired a series of later works in which the focus narrowed from the social to the purely sexual aspects. The still available and better known of these works are: the eleventh-century *Nagarasarvasva* of the Buddhist monk Padmashri; the twelfth-century *Ratirahasya* of Kokkoka from Kashmir; the fourteenth-century *Panchasayaka* of Jyotirisha, perhaps from Gujarat; the fifteenth-century *Ratiratnapradipika* of Praudha Devaraja from the south Indian Vijayanagara kingdom; and the sixteenth-century *Anangaranga* of Kalyanamalla, who wrote it for the Afghan chieftain Lad Khan Lodi. All except the last of these texts cite Vatsyayana, testifying to the currency of his work and reputation over more than a millennium. All are mainly elaborations of the *Kama Sutra*'s second book on sexual union, and some of them have also been cited by later writers. They include further classifications of male and female sexual types, new techniques of making love, cosmetic methods for beautification and theories linking erogenous zones of the female body with the phases of the moon.

The *Kama Sutra* also prompted learned commentaries on it in Sanskrit. The earliest known from quotation is the *Vatsyayana Sutrasara* of Kshemendra from eleventh-century Kashmir, but its text is lost. The most reputed now is the *Jayamangala*, composed in the thirteenth century by Yashodhara. Others include the sixteenth-century *Kandarpachudamani* by Virabhadra, actually a condensation of the *Kama Sutra* in verse; the unpublished eighteenth-century *Praudhapriya* of Bhaskara Nrisimha; and another by Malladeva, known only by the name. Commentaries have also been published in India in recent times, in Bengali, Hindi, Tamil and Telugu.[14] Perhaps the best known of these is the Hindi commentary of 1964 by Devadatta Shastri; another is the Hindi *Purusharthaprabha* by Madhavacharya, reprinted in 1995.

Translations into English

The first translation of the *Kama Sutra* into English appeared in 1883. It is still well known as the work of the explorer and linguist Sir Richard Burton, who also translated the *Arabian Nights*. Actually it was the result of a joint effort by him and another British colonial official, Foster Fitzgerald Arbuthnot, and two Indian scholars, Bhagvanlal Indraji and Shivaram Bhide, whom they had recruited for assistance in the translation. Published privately in view of the standards of censorship then prevailing, it soon acquired a reputation for pornography, leading to numerous pirated versions.[15]

Formally published in the United States and Britain only in 1962, the Burton translation still remains perhaps the most circulated of those in English. It has had several editions with learned comments by different scholars, and also been translated into other languages. Other translations into English have also appeared; some are listed in the Select Bibliography.

Recent scholarly translators have considered the Burton translation to be 'seriously flawed'.[16] A debate on this, as also on other translations, could possibly be of some academic interest, but this is not the place for it. Here it may suffice to touch briefly on translation in general and specially from Sanskrit.

An important aspect is the distinction between what may be called literal and literary translation. The first transmits information about meanings and the linguistic form in which they are presented: its main concern is fidelity to the original text, even if the readability of the rendition is thereby affected. It serves the academic purpose of better comprehending the original and its environment, and of facilitating further research. The second, on the other hand, is intended to bring the work to a more general readership through its own language. Apart from being accurate and readable, it needs to convey also a flavour and feel of the original. In the case of the *Kama Sutra*, with its compressed, aphoristic *sutra* form in Sanskrit, there is an additional need to make the language clearer through amplification. This necessitates consulting commentaries while taking care that they do not creep into the translation itself.

The Present Translation

The present translation is for the general reader interested in the *Kama Sutra* as it is. It refrains from extraneous comment and annotation more suited for the specialist, except where it may help better understanding of the original's language. I have endeavoured to combine faithfulness to the original text with the requirements of modern English usage. While using the Yashodhara and Shastri commentaries, which are much later and reflect their own times, to follow the text better, I have also tried to confine my translation to what Vatsyayana wrote, which is generally clear enough. I have further attempted to convey something of his dispassionate tone and occasional personal touch by translating his stanzas in a free verse form.

I have also avoided looking for any esoteric meanings which some suppose the text may contain, whether in its discussion of human relations or of sexual conduct. It touches on issues of current topicality like same-sex activities and trans-sexual behaviour, and what may be considered unorthodox practices. Some, like hitting and biting while making love and oral sex, are discussed in it at length while mention of others is marginal or incidental. In translating them I have followed the text as it is without any attempt at embellishment or interpretation. Clarifications of language, where they seemed needed, have been made in the notes to the text.

The *sutras* have been grouped in paragraphs for ease of reading. Their number from the text is given at the end of each paragraph for reference. The verses have been treated similarly.

The book and the chapter headings are translations from the text, but within each chapter I have inserted sub-headings for better reading. Thirty-two of these are based on Yashodhara's commentary; they are also mentioned in the text (1.1.15–22) but without indicating their placement as Yashodhara does. These sub-headings have been marked in the text with an asterisk. The others I have devised.

The text used for this translation is that published in 1964 by the Chaukhamba Sanskrit Sansthan, Varanasi, with the Sanskrit commentary *Jayamangala* of Yashodhara and the Hindi commentary of Devadatta Shastri. I have also compared it for corrections with the Sanskrit text brought out by Pratibha Prakashan, Delhi, in 2005 with English notes and translation by Radhavallabha Tripathi.

I am grateful to Penguin Classics and Marcella Edwards for asking me to undertake this new translation, and to Adam Freudenheim and Alexis Kirschbaum for giving me additional time to complete it. My gratitude also to Louise Willder, Anna Hervé and Linden Lawson for editing the copy. I am further obliged to Sushma Zutshi, Librarian of India International Centre, New Delhi, and her colleagues Shafali Bhatt and Rajeev Mishra for all their help with the reference material. Special thanks to my daughter-in-law Annika for her computer assistance at a crucial moment. Above all I thank my wife Priti for her patient and always helpful reading of the drafts and for her constant support and encouragement, which I cannot describe in words. This work is dedicated to her on our wedding anniversary today.

A.N.D.H.
Noida, Uttar Pradesh
19 November 2010

BOOK ONE
General

CHAPTER ONE:

Summary of the Work

Salutations

Reverence to Dharma, Artha and Kama, the subjects of this work, and to the teachers who expounded their principles and their relationship.
(1–4)

History

After creating mankind, for the basis of its existence the Lord of Beings first enunciated in one hundred thousand chapters the means for pursuing the aforementioned three ends of life in this world.
(5)

Manu, the son of the self-born Lord, segregated one part of these into a separate work about Dharma, that is virtuous conduct, and Brihaspati did the same with another part concerning Artha, or material gain.
(6–7)

The great god's servant Nandi separated Kama Sutra, the precepts on pleasure, and put them forth in one thousand chapters. These were compressed by Shvetaketu, the son of Uddalaka, into five hundred chapters, and Babhravya of Panchala abridged them further to one hundred and fifty chapters in seven books: General,

Sexual Union, the Maiden, the Wife, the Wives of Others, the Courtesan and Esoteric Matters.
(8–10)

From the sixth of these books, the Courtesan, Dattaka composed a separate work at the behest of the elite courtesans of Pataliputra. In the same way, Charayana separately expounded the book General; Suvarnanabha that on Sexual Union; Ghotakamukha on the Maiden; Gonardiya on the Wife; Gonikaputra on the Wives of Others; and Kuchumara on Esoteric Matters.
(11–12)

Thus presented piecemeal by many teachers, the work itself virtually disappeared. The expositions of Dattaka and the others were merely parts of the same body of knowledge, and that of Babhravya was difficult to study because of its great length. The present *Kama Sutra*, Vatsyayana says, is offered after condensing all the material in one brief volume.
(13–14)

Contents

Here is an account of the books and the chapters in this work. The first book, entitled General, consists of five chapters and subjects: Summary of the Work; Achieving the Three Ends; The Arts Outlined; The Gentleman's Life; and The Work of Helpers and Messengers.
(15–16)

The second book, Sexual Union, has ten chapters dealing with seventeen subjects: Kinds of Union; Types of Pleasure; Embracing; Kissing; Scratching; Biting; Regional Practices; Methods of Intercourse; Unusual Sex; Hitting; Moaning;

Reversing Roles; The Male Approach; Oral Sex; Before and After; Kinds of Sex; and Lovers' Quarrels.

(17)

The third book, on The Maiden, has five chapters covering nine subjects: Arranging a Marriage; A Decisive Point; Winning the Girl's Trust; Approaching a Maiden; Her Responses; The Man's Advances; The Woman's Advances; Winning the Maiden; and Other Types of Marriage.

(18)

The fourth book, The Wife, has two chapters on eight subjects: The Only Wife; Conduct in the Husband's Absence; The Senior Wife; The Junior Wife; The Remarried Woman; The Unlucky Wife; Life in the Harem; and The Man with Several Wives.

(19)

The fifth book, on Wives of Others, has six chapters concerning ten subjects: The Nature of Women and Men; Why Women Get Turned Off; Overcoming Resistance; Easy Women; Gaining Access; Making a Pass; Appraisal of Feelings; The Go-Between's Role; Sex and Men in Power; and Guarding the Harem.

(20)

The sixth book, The Courtesan, comprises six chapters on twelve subjects: Worthwhile and Avoidable Clients; Motivations; Getting a Client; Pleasing the Lover; Making Money; Signs of the Lover Cooling Off; Getting Him Back; Getting Rid of Him; Reunion with an ex-Lover; Particular Profits; Gains and Losses, Consequences and Doubts; and Kinds of Courtesan.

(21)

The seventh book, Esoteric Matters, has two chapters on six subjects: Looking Good; Bewitching a Woman; Enhancing

Virility; Revival of Passion; Enlarging the Penis; and Various Prescriptions.
(22)

Thus there are thirty-six chapters dealing with sixty-four subjects in these seven books, which comprise one and a quarter thousand precepts in all. This concludes the summary of the work.
(23)

> This brief accounting
> will now be expanded,
> for the wise of this world like statements
> to be detailed as well as summary.
> (24)

CHAPTER TWO:

Achieving the Three Ends

The Suitable Age

Man has a lifespan of one hundred years. This time should be parcelled out in so pursuing the three ends of life, which are interconnected, that they do not interfere with each other. Early life is the time for acquiring knowledge and other material things. Youth is for pleasure, and old age is a time for the pursuit of virtue and salvation. However, as the span of life is uncertain, one should pursue whatever is achievable. But celibacy should be observed while one is a student acquiring knowledge.
(1–6)

Dharma

Dharma is action and abstention in accordance with the rules. It is, for example, the engagement in sacred sacrificial and other rituals, even by those disinclined towards them because these works are other-worldly and their results cannot be seen; and the avoidance, even by those given to them, of eating meat and suchlike, which are worldly activities with visible results. Dharma can be learnt from the revealed scriptures and by association with people who understand it.
(7–8)

Artha

Artha is the acquisition of knowledge, land, cattle, gold, grain, household goods, friends and so forth; and the enhancement of what has been acquired. It can be learnt from the conduct of eminent people and from those knowledgeable about professions and conventions, agriculture and trade.
(9–10)

Kama

Kama is the mind's inclination towards objects which a person's senses of hearing, touch, sight, taste and smell find congenial. Its principal element is a delightful, creative feeling pervaded by sensual pleasure and derived in particular from

the sense of touch. It should be learnt from the *Kama Sutra* and from association with civilized people.
(11–13)

Comparing the Three Ends

Considered together, Dharma is more important than Artha, and Artha more than Kama. But Artha can be more important for the king, and also for the courtesan, as it is the basis of worldly life.
(14–15)

It is appropriate to have a work explaining Dharma as it is other-worldly, and another for making known the means for achieving Artha. On the other hand, according to many teachers, Kama needs no treatise as it is eternal and comes naturally, even to animals. However, woman and man depend on each other in sexual union and they need knowledge of the methods. These, says Vatsyayana, are available in the *Kama Sutra*. Animals do not need them as they are devoid of inhibition and their sexual inclination is determined by the female's fertile period without any prior thought.
(16–20)

Questions and Answers

Why pursue Dharma? Its fruit lies in future lives and then too is uncertain. Which wise person will give away something in hand to someone else? A pigeon today is better than a peacock tomorrow and, as the materialists say, an authentic copper penny is better than a doubtful coin of gold.
(21–24)

Vatsyayana says that the scriptures are beyond doubt. Their rituals are also seen to bear fruit from time to time. The heavenly constellations, the sun and the moon, the stars and the planets, display in their movements a deliberate concern for the world. Stability in worldly existence is marked by the observance of the rules concerning the classes and the stages of life. Worldly existence also demonstrates that the seed in hand is given up for the sake of a future crop. As such, Dharma should be followed

(25)

Why pursue Artha? Sometimes it cannot be achieved even with effort, and occasionally it comes on its own. As the fatalists say, all things are fated. Fate alone causes gain and loss, victory and defeat, comfort and distress. Destiny alone raised Bali to the position of Indra, again cast him down and may elevate him once more.

(26–29)

But all activity presupposes effort and method, says Vatsyayana. Even inevitable results require them. So, no good can come to one who does nothing.

(30–31)

Why pursue Kama? Those who are prudent say it is an obstacle to Dharma and Artha, which are more important. It obstructs virtuous company and leads man into association with worthless people, wicked practices, impurity and bad consequences. It also makes one careless. No one respects, believes or accepts such a person. It is said that under the influence of Kama many have perished along with their families, like the Bhoja ruler Dandakya who lusted for a brahmin's daughter and was destroyed together with his clan and kingdom. The same was the case of the king of the gods with Ahalya, the mighty Kichaka with Draupadi, Ravana with Sita, and many others.

(32–36)

Vatsyayana says that Kama, like food, is a means for the body's sustenance. It is also a fruit of Dharma and Artha. Its shortcomings should be taken into account, but will one not eat food because there are beggars who need it, or not sow seeds because there are beasts who may eat the crop? There are some verses on this:
(37–38)

One who thus pursues
Artha, Kama and Dharma
enjoys untroubled happiness
in this world and the next
(39)

Civilized folk will act in ways
that give pleasure, but do no harm
to the end of material gain
nor cause worry about results
of their deeds in the world hereafter.
Their actions should be for achieving
all the three ends of human life,
or just two or even one,
but not to obstruct two of them
in pursuit of a single end.
(40)

CHAPTER THREE:
The Arts Outlined

Their Study

A man should study the *Kama Sutra* and its subsidiary subjects without detracting from his time for Dharma, Artha and the subjects related to them. A woman should study it too before she reaches the prime of her youth. If married, she should do so with her husband's consent.
(1–2)

Learning and Women

Some teachers say that instructing women in this knowledge is meaningless as they cannot comprehend science. But women understand application, says Vatsyayana, and that depends on science. This is also not unique. All over the world the knowledge of science is limited to a few people but its application concerns everyone. And, though science may be far removed from application, it is still the latter's source.
(3–6)

Take grammar. Even priests who do not know it as a science use it in sacrificial incantations. The same is the case with astronomy and the determination of auspicious days for the performance of sacred rituals. Similarly, syces and mahouts train horses and elephants without having studied the respective sciences; and people do not transgress the king's law even though he may be far away.
(7–10)

It is the same with women and the science of pleasure. Indeed there are elite courtesans, royal princesses and high officials' daughters with minds well honed by it. A woman should therefore learn the science and its application, or at least a part of it, from some trustworthy persons in private.
(11–12)

The Training of Girls

The sixty-four arts require training for their application, and a maiden should also practise them privately by herself. Her teachers can be: her wet-nurse's daughter, who has grown up with her and is already experienced in sex with a man; a similarly experienced girl friend who will speak to her without reserve; a maternal aunt of her own age; an old maidservant who is equally reliable; a nun well known to her; and her own sister, if she has her confidence in such matters.
(13–14)

The Sixty-four Arts

These are the sixty-four subsidiary subjects for study with the *Kama Sutra*:

Singing; instrumental music; dancing; painting; cutting leaves into special shapes for use as beauty spots; making decorative patterns with rice grains and flowers; arranging flowers; colouring the teeth, the body and garments; inlaying gems in floors; making beds; making music with bowls of water; splashing water in games; various cures; stringing garlands; making diadems and chaplets; fancy dress costumes; making ear ornaments;

mixing perfumes; arrangement of jewellery; conjuring tricks; casting spells; sleights of hand; preparation of unusual vege- tables, soups and other things to eat; preparation of juices, wines and other things to drink; needlework; weaving tricks; playing the lute and the drum; telling and solving riddles; capping words; reciting difficult verses; reading aloud; staging plays and stories; completing stanzas; making things from cloth, cane and straw; enamelwork; wood-carving; architecture; assessment of gems, metallurgy; knowledge of colours and sources of gems; horticulture; setting up fights between rams, cocks and quails; teaching parrots and mynah birds to talk; skills of cleaning, mas- saging and hair-dressing; speaking in sign language; use of secret words; knowledge of dialects; making flower toys; knowledge of omens; making magical diagrams; the art of memorization; repeating heard phrases or verses; improvisation of poetry; knowledge of dictionaries; knowledge of prosody; knowledge of poetics; mimicry; using clothes for disguise; special types of gambling; games with the dice; children's games; knowledge of etiquette; knowledge of strategic sciences; knowledge of ath- letic skills. The sixty-four arts of Panchala are different. They are erotic in nature and we will speak of their application in the book on sexual union.

(15–16)

The Benefits of Learning

A public woman who excels
in these arts, and is possessed
of character, good looks and merit,
wins the name 'elite courtesan'
and a place in people's assemblies.

Always honoured by the king
and praised by men of quality,
she becomes a focal point
for requests and supplications
and intimate approaches.
(17–18)
A princess or a minister's daughter
who knows these arts can win control
of her husband, even though
his harem have a thousand women.
And, separated from her lord,
fallen into dire straits,
even in a foreign land,
with these skills she will be able
still to lead a life of comfort.
(19–20)
And, in these arts adept, a man
who's good with words and flattery,
will quickly win the hearts of women –
a stranger to them though he may be.
(21)
Luck in love can come about
with just a knowledge of these arts.
But one must also take account
of time and place to see if they
can be put to use or not.
(22)

CHAPTER FOUR:

The Gentleman's Life

His Abode

After getting educated one should set up as a householder, using the money one has acquired either through inheritance or through gifts, conquest, trade and wages, or by both means. One can then live the life of a gentleman. This can be in a metropolis, a city or a large market town, wherever good people live or travel takes one. Have a house built there. It should be near water, have an orchard and separate quarters for working, and contain two bedrooms.
(1–3)

The outer bedroom should have a good soft bed, low in the middle, with two pillows and a white sheet spread over it. At its head there is a place for a brush and a stand for keeping a pot of beeswax, a bottle of perfume, some lemon peel and betel leaves. Creams and garlands left over from the night before can also be placed there. On the ground is a spittoon. A lute hangs from a peg of ivory on the wall. Near it there is a drawing board with pencils, a book and a garland of amaranth leaves.
(4)

A couch is kept near the bed, and not too far from it a round, cushioned seat spread on the ground with dice and gambling boards on it. Outside the bedroom are cages for pet birds, and a secluded place for wood-carving and other pastimes. In the orchard there is a padded swing in the shade and a bench of baked clay spread with flowers.
(4 continued)

His Daily Routine

After getting up in the morning and relieving himself a gentle-man cleans his teeth and rubs some scented paste on his body. Perfuming his hair with incense smoke, applying beeswax and red lac to his face and putting on a garland, he then looks at himself in a mirror and freshens his mouth with betel leaf before attending to the day's work.
(5)

He should bathe every day, have a massage every second day and use the fish-bone body-scraper every third day. The nails and the whiskers should be trimmed every fourth day and the body hair removed every fifth or tenth day. The armpits should always be kept clean of perspiration.
(6)

He should eat in the morning and the afternoon. In the even-ing too, according to Charayana. After meals he spends time making his parrots and mynah birds talk, watching quail, cock and ram fights and other similar recreation. He also interacts with his companions, parasites and jesters, and then has a nap.
(7–8)

By the late afternoon he is dressed to go out for social gath-erings and soirées. At dusk there are concerts of music. After that he returns to his chamber, which has meanwhile been dec-orated and perfumed with incense smoke, and waits there by the bedside with his aides for girlfriends coming out to meet him. A messenger woman may be sent to fetch them or he may go himself.
(9–11)

When they arrive he and his aides should receive them with all courtesies and many winning words. If they have come in

bad weather and their clothes have got wet in the rain, he should himself redo their makeup or have his friends attend to this. Such is his routine, by day and night.
(12–13)

His Diversions

A gentleman may amuse himself by going to festivals, soirées, drinking parties, picnics and literary games.
(14)

Festivals

As for these, there is always a gathering of select people at the temple of the goddess Sarasvati on a specified day every month or fortnight. Actors and dancers perform there. Also visiting artists, who receive appropriate prizes on the following day and are asked to stay on or dismissed depending on the audience's reaction. Both groups should naturally work together during the festival, as well as in any trouble. It is their duty to honour and help other visitors and outsiders. Such festivals also take place at other temples dedicated to particular deities.
(15–18)

Soirées

A soirée or social gathering may take place at the house of a courtesan, an assembly hall or an individual's dwelling place. On such occasions people of the same age, with similar education and intelligence, means and inclinations, get together for congenial conversation and discussion of questions of poetry and art with courtesans. Like-minded ones are brought to these gatherings and the brilliant and popular among them are specially honoured.

(19–21)

Drinking Parties

Drinking parties are held at one another's houses. There courtesans ply guests with wines and spirits made from honey, molasses, grain and fruit, and also drink with them. They further serve them relishes, salty and spicy, bitter and sour, with fruit, greens and vegetables.

(22–23)

Picnics

Picnics in parks and gardens can be described in the same way. Dressed with care and mounted on horseback, men go out in the morning. They are accompanied by courtesans and followed by servants. These are day trips. The participants spend time betting on cock fights, watching theatrical shows and in other agreeable activities. They return in the evening, carrying souvenirs of their pleasures in the park. In the summer they go similarly for water sports in pools and tanks filled artificially.

(24–26)

Games

These include goblin nights, moonlit wakes, spring festivals and well-known games peculiar to different regions, like plucking the mango, eating roasted grain, nibbling lotus stems, collecting new leaves, squirting water, pantomimes, the silk-cotton tree game and mock-fights with wild jasmine flowers. People play them as they wish. A solitary man can also play depending on his means, and so can courtesans and other women with their girlfriends and other men.
(27–30)

His Aides

One is called the companion. He has no wealth, only himself. A wooden seat, a back-scraper and some astringent are his sole possessions. But he hails from a respectable background, is skilled in all the arts and makes a living by teaching them at social gatherings, together with proper manners for courtesans. Another is called the parasite. He had wealth but has used it up. A married person of quality, he subsists on the general reputation he has among courtesans and assemblies. Then there is the jester or clown. His knowledge is limited, but he is good company and completely trustworthy. These are the people courtesans and gentlemen use as advisers in their compacts and disputes, as they do skilled beggar women, unmarried girls, widows and old courtesans.
(31–35)

The Rural Gentleman

A gentleman living in a village should describe the cultured life of the city to intelligent and curious members of his community and encourage their desire to live similarly. He should arrange social gatherings with these people, give them entertaining company, help them in their work and earn their gratitude by doing them favours. So much for the life of a gentleman. (36)

Some Dos and Don'ts

In gatherings, to gain esteem
and respect among the people,
do not talk too much in Sanskrit
nor too much in the local language.
(37)

The wise will not attend
a gathering unpopular,
which is but a free-for-all
and causes hurt to others.
(38)

But one which is in keeping
with the public mood, and whose
sole function is amusement:
by going to such gatherings
the wise attain success.
(39)

CHAPTER FIVE:

The Work of Helpers and Messengers

Rules for Sex

The law books sanction sex with a woman of the same caste, one who has not been with another man before, as the source of progeny, good reputation and social acceptability. Contrary to it is sex with a woman of a higher caste or one who is another's wife. Sex with a woman of a lower caste or an outcaste is also prohibited. But with a courtesan and a previously married woman it is neither recommended nor proscribed, as then it is purely for pleasure.
(1–2)

Permissible Women and Adultery

Women with whom one may sleep are thus of three kinds: a virgin girl, a previously married woman and a courtesan.
(3)

  A fourth kind, according to Gonikaputra, can optionally even be one married to another man, but this depends on particular reasons. For example, she may already be known as a loose woman robbed of her virtue by many others. So, even though she is of a higher caste, sleeping with her is like with a courtesan or a previously married woman, and will not go against Dharma. Thus there should be no hesitation in this case as she has already been had before.
(4–7)

A variation may concern the woman's husband. 'He is a great lord,' one may consider, 'and he is partial to someone who is my enemy. She has influence over him and, on becoming my intimate, she can turn him against that person out of love for me.' Or, 'her husband has the ability to harm me and now seems set to do so as he has turned hostile. She can improve his attitude towards me.' Or, 'winning his friendship through her, I will be able to help my comrades, repel my foes or accomplish some other difficult task.' Or even, 'after becoming her lover, I will be able to kill her spouse and get hold of the treasure which should have been mine.'
(8–11)

Or, one may reason, 'there is no sin in sleeping with her as I have no money, few means of livelihood, and in this way stand to gain enormous wealth without any difficulty.' Or, 'she is infatuated with me and also knows my secrets. If I do not respond to her passion, she will make my faults public and bring me into disrepute.' Or, 'she will accuse me of some grave misdemeanour, which is baseless but difficult to disprove, so that I am ruined.'
(12–14)

Or one may think, 'her husband is influential but also under her control. She can turn him against me and towards my adversaries.' Or, 'she may herself join them.' Or, 'her husband violated my harem, so my violation of his women is no more than revenge.'
(15–16)

Or, 'in keeping with a royal directive, I will be able to destroy the king's enemy who is hiding inside her house.' Or, 'with her co-operation I will be able to possess another woman whom I desire and who is under her influence.' Or, 'she can get me a rich, beautiful and otherwise unattainable virgin girl who

depends on her.' Or, 'through her I can plan to poison my enemy who is a boon companion of her husband.'
(17–20)

For such reasons as the above, one may even sleep with another man's wife. But such a rash step should never be taken just out of passion alone. So much for the grounds for adultery.
(20–21)

For the same reasons, according to Charayana, there is a fifth kind of woman permissible for sex: a widow related to a high official, to the king, or to their families or another who can get things done. A sixth, according to Suvarnanabha, is the female ascetic. A seventh, Ghotakamukha says, is an elite courtesan's daughter or girl attendant, neither of whom has had a man before. And Gonardiya says that an eighth kind is a mature young woman from a good family, as she needs a different approach. But, in the absence of any real differences, all these women actually come under the earlier classification. And that, according to Vatsyayana, is just four kinds of women permissible for sexual relations. The fifth kind, some believe, is a person of the third nature. But that is different.
(22–27)

The Lovers

As for the lovers of these women, one is the kind known to all. The second is the secret lover seeking some special benefit. They can be classified further as the best, the worst and the middling, depending on their qualities or lack of them. We will speak about the virtues and defects of both in the book on courtesans.
(28)

Forbidden Women

The following women are proscribed for sexual relations: a leper, a lunatic, a fallen woman, a betrayer of secrets, one who solicits openly, one past her prime, one too fair or too dark, a malodorous woman, a relative, a colleague, a nun, and the wives of relatives, friends, priests and kings.
(29)

According to the followers of Babhravya, any woman who has already had five men cannot be proscribed. But Gonikaputra still excludes from this list the wives of relatives, friends, priests and kings.
(30–31)

Helpers

A friend is one who has played with you in the dust as a child, one of similar character and defects, a classmate, one whose secrets and weaknesses you know and who knows yours, and one who has the same foster mother and has grown up with you. His father and grandfather were friends with yours. He keeps his word, is constant, steadfast and dependent on you. He is not greedy, will not betray confidences or be turned against you. These are what make a friend.
(32–33)

According to Vatsyayana, a gentleman's friends can be laundrymen, barbers, florists, perfumers, vintners, beggars, cowherds, betel-sellers and goldsmiths, as well as his companions, parasites and jesters, and their women.
(34)

Messengers

One who relates to both partners, and is open-minded towards both, specially the woman: such a person can be used with confidence as a messenger. The qualities desirable in such a person are eloquence, pertness, an understanding of the signals of emotion, a knowledge of the right time for deception, a feel for what is possible, quick grasp and resourcefulness. (35–36)

> A man who is self-confident,
> possessed of friends and diligent too,
> understands the time and the place,
> and the other person's feelings,
> can win over, with no effort,
> even women hard to get.
> (37)

BOOK TWO

Sexual Union

CHAPTER ONE:

Kinds of Union

By Size

In keeping with the size of their sex organs, from the small to
the middling and the large, men are typed as the hare, the bull
and the horse; and women as the doe, the mare and the elephant
woman.
(1)

Thus there are three equal unions in sex, where the partners
are of the same size. On the other hand, there are six unequal
unions. Two of these, where the man is larger than the two
women next in size, are known as 'the high'; and another,
where he is larger still, as 'the highest'. On the other hand,
there are two unions called 'the low', and another, of the small-
est man with the largest woman, called 'the lowest'.
(2–3)

Of all these unions, the equal ones are the best and the highest and the lowest the least good. The rest are middling unions,
though in them too it is better for the man to be larger than the
woman, rather than the other way round. In sum, there are
nine types of union according to size.
(4)

By Temperament

While making love, if a man is indifferent to the pleasure, has little virility and cannot bear to be hurt, his sexual impulse is classed as dull. By the same criteria there are men with middling or intense sexual impulses. With women, too, it is the same. Thus, here also there are nine kinds of sexual union, just as in the earlier classification by size.
(5–7)

By Duration

In duration, similarly, there are men who climax quickly, those who are middling in this respect and those who can carry on for long. But the case of women is debatable on this point.
(8–9)

Questions of Climax

In the view of Auddalaki, a woman does not climax like a man. She has an itch which gets relieved by the man's continued friction inside her. Combined with the erotic arousal of foreplay, this generates a different kind of feeling in her sense of pleasure.
(10–12)

How can pleasure be determined, it may be asked. Man and woman cannot know what it is like in the other, nor can they ask how it is. The answer, says Auddalaki, is that the man stops

on his own after reaching a climax and pays no attention to the woman. With her it is different. Women, it should be noted, love the man who can continue for long and dislike one who finishes quickly, as they are then unable to reach their own climax at the end. Both these reactions are signs of their having achieved a climax or not.
(13–15)

It can be argued that these signs are ambiguous. What is evident, however, is that even relieving the itch for a long duration can be pleasurable:
(16–17)

> A woman's itch obtains relief
> in her union with a man
> and that, combined with love's foreplay,
> is what is called her sexual pleasure.
> (16–17)

According to the followers of Babhravya, a young woman has a continuing emotional climax from the beginning of intercourse. A man reaches it only as he concludes. It is, they say, well known that conception is not possible without her achieving a climax.
(18)

But here too there are doubts needing resolution. Thus, at the commencement of sex the woman's mindset may be indifferent, with not much tolerance of pain. Gradually her passion increases and she no longer cares for her body. At the end she wants to stop. All this is evident and cannot be reconciled with any continuity of climax. Even in ordinary motion, for example the revolution of a potter's wheel or the spinning of a top, the movement is slow in the beginning, attains full momentum by degrees and tends to stop as that dissipates. This is irrefutable:

> But they say man's bliss
> comes with his climax,
> and for a woman
> it is continuous –
> her wish to conclude
> is caused by dissipation
> of bodily fluids.
> (19–22)

According to Vatsyayana, orgasm is as manifest in the woman as in the man. How can there be a difference in the end sought by two persons of the same species engaged in the same endeavour? There may be differences in approach and in feeling. The former are due to physical nature. The man is the active doer, the girl a passive recipient. The doer contributes to action in one way, the recipient in another. And from this physical difference comes the difference in feeling. The man is aroused by the thought 'I am possessing her', and the girl by the thought 'I am being possessed by him'.
(23–26)

It may be objected that if there is a difference in approach, it should also be there in the end sought. But it is not so. The approach has a cause, that is the different characteristics of the doer and the recipient. But there is no cause to establish any difference in the end sought by two persons of the same species.
(27)

It may also be objected that this analogy is inappropriate. While a work done jointly produces a single end, here two persons are intent on achieving their separate ends. However, even this does not hold. Two actions can achieve a single goal, as one may see in the clash of two rams in a contest, the striking-together of two wood-apples and the grapple of two wrestlers. To the comment that there is no distinction between the actors in these cases, it can be said that there is no essential distinction in the case of man and woman either. The difference in their approaches, as already stated, is due to their physical makeup. But their experience of pleasure is the same:

> The couple are of the same species,
> the pleasure they seek is the same.
> But the woman should be handled so
> that she reaches her climax first.
> (28–30)

Pleasure in Sex

The similarity of a couple's pleasure has thus been established. In terms of duration and endurance also there are nine kinds of sexual union, as there are by temperament and size.
(31)

Erotic feeling, delight, pleasure, loving emotion, sexual impulse and consummation: these are the stages of *rati* or bliss during sexual union. The stages of the union itself, of *rata*, are: coming together, coupling, privacy, going to bed together and intercourse.
(32)

Given that there are nine kinds of sexual union in keeping with the criteria of size, duration and temperament, it is not possible to enumerate all their combinations, which are far too many. Vatsyayana says they should be chosen and used with due care.
(33–34)

The man's impulse is intense but his endurance brief in the first coupling; in later ones it is the opposite. For women it is the other way round, until the fluid gets discharged. Also, it is often said that the man's fluid gets discharged before the woman's.

> The scholars are agreed
> that women climax quicker,
> being delicate by nature,
> if they are aroused.
> (35–37)

Types of Pleasure*

> So far, sexual union has
> been spoken of for expert minds;
> now it is elaborated
> to enlighten the dull.
> (38)

> Knowers of the science say
> that pleasure is of four sorts:
> that which comes from habit, or
> from arousal or belief
> or from sense perceptions.
> (39)

> Pleasure from habit is seen
> in several habitual actions
> like hunting and others
> not manifest in words.
> (40)

Pleasure from arousal
is engendered in the mind,
not in previous habit
or any sense perception.
(41)

It is there in kissing
and other such activities,
in oral sex with women
or persons who are eunuchs.
(42)

When the thought
'He is not different'
causes pleasure in another:
those who know the science
call it pleasure from belief.
(43)

Pleasure from sense perceptions
is there for all to see.
Its result is the best of all
and the other three seek it too.
(44)

Considering all these pleasures,
and in keeping with the scriptures
where they are characterized,
one should act in such a way
as will suit one's feelings.
(45)

CHAPTER TWO:

Embracing

The Theory of Sixty-four

It is said that sexual union has sixty-four elements. Some teachers call the science of sex itself 'the sixty-four' as it is recounted in that number of chapters. Or, as there are sixty-four arts associated with sexual union, the number may refer to this aggregate. Just as the verses of the *Rigveda*, being grouped in ten sections, are sometimes called 'the ten', here too a similar meaning may have been derived. Some scholars say that the title has been used to honour its connection with the sage Panchala who divided the verses in this number.
(1–3)

The followers of Babhravya hold that the number derives from eight times eight. Sexual union has eight parts: embracing, kissing, scratching, biting, coition, moaning, reversing roles and oral sex, and each of these has eight varieties. But these can also be more or less than eight. Besides this, there are other parts like hitting, screaming, the male approach and unusual sex. So 'sixty-four' is just an expression, according to Vatsyayana, like a 'seven-leaf' tree or a 'five-colour' sacrificial offering.
(4–5)

Indicators of Readiness

For a couple yet to make
love together, there are four

embraces which convey
their pleasure in each other:
the touch, the thrust and then the rub,
and one called the hard embrace.
(6)

In each case the name itself denotes the action. Thus, the woman a man wants is before him. He passes by her and under some pretext brushes his body against hers. This is 'the touch'. (7–8)

The man a woman wants is sitting or standing alone. Pretending that she is carrying something, she pushes him with her breasts and he holds her close. This is 'the thrust'. Both these embraces are for couples who have yet to speak freely with each other.
(9–10)

When a couple are walking slowly in the dark, in a crowd, or in a lonely place, they rub their bodies against each other for not too short a time. This is 'the rub'. And when they press each other hard against a wall or a pillar, it is called 'the hard embrace'. These two are for couples who understand each other's intentions.
(11–13)

Preludes to Sex

There are four embraces at the time of actual sexual union: the 'twining creeper', the 'climbing a tree', the 'sesame seeds and rice grains' and the 'milk and water'.
(14)

The 'twining creeper' is now described. She twines herself

around him like a vine around the *sala* tree, and draws his face down to kiss him. Then, raising it gently, she sighs, leaning against him and looking at him lovingly. The 'climbing a tree' has her placing one foot over his with her other leg across his thigh or wrapped around him. With one arm clasping his back and the other tugging at his shoulders, she pants and moans, wanting as if to climb him for a kiss. Both these embraces are done while standing up.
(15–17)

Lying on a bed, their thighs and arms entwined, the couple hold each other tightly, as if wrestling. This is the 'sesame and rice'. And she sits facing him, on his lap or on the bed. Then, blind with passion and heedless of pain, they want to reach as far inside each other as possible. This is called the 'milk and water'. Both are for intense moments of passion.
(18–20)

These are the embraces mentioned by the followers of Babhravya. Suvarnanabha has added four more for specific parts of the body.
(21–22)

The thighs are used like a pair of tongs to squeeze one or both thighs of the other, with all one's might. This is called the 'embrace of the thighs'. And, pressing his pelvis against hers, her massed hair flowing, she straddles across him, to scratch and bite, strike and kiss him. This is the 'pelvic embrace'.
(23–24)

The 'embrace of the breasts' is accomplished by her thrusting both her breasts on to his chest so that their weight bears down upon him. And to press against each other, mouth to mouth, eyes to eyes, forehead to forehead, is called the 'forehead embrace'.
(25–26)

Massage

Some consider massage also to be a kind of embrace as it involves touching. But Vatsyayana disagrees as it has a separate time and a different purpose; moreover, it may not be enjoyed by both parties in the same way.
(27–28)

Summation

This is the way of deep embraces.
Even those who ask about it,
or listen to it being talked of,
or explain the whole of it,
are actually wanting to make love.
Some other ways not prescribed here
also serve to build up passion.
They too may be used in love
but only with due care.
For prescriptions are relevant only
till men's feelings dull remain.
Once the wheel of bliss erotic
is in motion, there is neither
prescription nor any order.
(29–31)

CHAPTER THREE:

Kissing

The Occasions

There is no particular order in kissing, scratching and biting as they are all manifestations of passion. They are used mainly before sexual union, and striking and moaning during intercourse. According to Vatsyayana all of them can be used at any time as passion knows no order. However, during the first union with a trusting woman, they should be used in slow degrees and not too blatantly. Once her passion is aroused, to further inflame it they can be used more rapidly and sometimes in unison. (1–3)

Spots for Kissing

The places for kissing are: the forehead, the hair, the cheeks, the eyes, the chest, the breasts, the hips and the inside of the mouth. The people of Lata also kiss on the place where the thigh joins the body, the armpit and the pudendum. But passion and local practice account for these spots, and they are not for everyone, says Vatsyayana. (4–6)

Raising the Pitch

There are three types of kisses for a virgin girl: the nominal, the throbbing and the brushing kiss. The first is when, forced to kiss the man, she places her mouth on his but stays motionless. A little less shy, when she wants to grasp the lip thrust forward into her mouth but only quivers her lower lip for this without daring to move the upper one, it is the throbbing kiss. In the brushing kiss, she shuts her eyes and covers his with her hands as she holds his lips gently between her own and brushes them with the tip of her tongue.

(7–10)

There are four other kisses: from the front, from the side, from the back and the hard kiss. A fifth one consists of bunching the other's lips with one's fingers into a ball and kissing them hard without using the teeth. This is the pressing kiss.

(11–12)

A Kissing Game

One can wager on kisses. Whichever of the partners first gets to the other's lower lip wins. If the woman loses, she sobs and flings out her hand, pushes the man off, bites him and turns her face away. If forced back, she starts arguing and demands another wager. And if she loses once more, she fusses twice as much again. If the man becomes too credulous or careless, she gets to his lower lip and catches it between her teeth so that it cannot be extricated. Then she laughs and shouts, taunts him, swaggers and exults, arches her brows and rolls her eyes, saying whatever she may please. This is the kissing wager and quarrel.

(13–16)

It is the same with mock-quarrels about scratching, biting and striking. But they are only for couples with sexual urges of similar intensity.

(17–18)

Special Kisses

If she is kissing his lower lip, he can grasp her upper one. This is the upper lip kiss.
(19)

Or he may kiss both her lips, pinching them together with his own. This is the clasping kiss. It can also be given by women to men whose whiskers have yet to sprout. In its course the tongue can be rubbed over the other's teeth, palate and tongue. This is the battle of the tongues, which may also be forcefully grasped by or thrust into the other's mouth between the teeth.
(20–22)

On other parts of the body, the kiss may be hard or gentle, with lips kept straight or pouted, depending on the spot. Such are the special kisses.
(23)

Signalling Desire

When she gazes at the sleeping man's mouth and kisses it on her own, it is called the kiss that kindles passion.
(24)

When he is inattentive or argumentative, looking at something else or dozing with his face turned away, the kiss to wake him up is known as the turn-on kiss.
(25)

When he comes in late at night, she is asleep in bed and he kisses her on his own, it is the awakening kiss. Of course, she

may only be pretending to sleep because she knows her lover has arrived and wants to gauge his mood.
(26–27)

Kissing the other's shadow or reflection in a mirror, on a wall or in water is also a way of making one's feelings known. So too the transferred kiss or embrace given to a child, a picture or a statue.
(28–29)

At night, during a performance or a family gathering, the man may get close to the woman and kiss her fingers or sit down and kiss her toes. Or, while massaging the man, she may signal to him by resting her head on his thighs as if she has no wish but to sleep, and then kiss them. Thus are advances made.
(30–31)

Summation

There is a verse that sums up all of this:

> Do what is done to you,
> hit back if you are hit;
> and, in the same way,
> if you are kissed, kiss back.
> (32)

CHAPTER FOUR:

Scratching

The Purpose and Places

Mounting passion is the time for rubbing and scratching each other with the fingernails. This can be done during the first intercourse, on return from or departure for a long journey, and with a woman propitiated after a tantrum or one who is drunk. But not every time, nor by couples whose sexual impulse is not intense. The same goes for biting by those with similar tastes.
(1–3)

Eight kinds of marks are made with fingernails: the 'mixed', the 'half-moon', the 'circle', the 'line', the 'tiger's claw', the 'peacock's foot', the 'leaping hare' and the 'lotus leaf'. The places for making them are: the armpits, the breasts, the neck, the back, the thighs and the pelvic area. But, as Suvarnanabha has said, once the wheel of sexual bliss has begun to turn there is no such thing as a place or non-place.
(4–6)

Kinds of Nail

Couples with intense sexual impulses should keep the nails of their left hands freshly trimmed with two or three points. Nails of good quality are clear and even, bright and clean, whole and growing, soft and glossy in appearance.
(7–8)

44

The people of Gauda have long fingernails which embellish their hands and capture the hearts of the women who see them. The southern people have short nails suited for work and for making whatever kinds of marks they choose. The qualities of both are found in the medium-sized nails of the people of Maharashtra.
(9–11)

Types of Scratch

When the nails are rubbed together to make a sound and the chin, the breasts or the lower lip are caressed with them so softly that no mark is left but the mere touch causes goose-pimples, it is called the 'mixed' scratch. It can be done on a woman while massaging her body or rubbing her head, squeezing her pimples or alarming her with something scary.
(12–13)

Curved marks made with the nails on the neck and the upper part of the breast are called the 'half-moon'. Two of these made face-to-face form the 'circle'. These are applied to the pudendum, the declivities of the bottom, and where the thighs meet the torso.
(14–16)

The 'line' mark can be applied everywhere, but it should not be too long. When it is curved and made at the front of the breast, it is called the 'tiger's claw'. When made with all the five nails around the nipple, it is the 'peacock's foot'. Five of these made around the nipple of a woman wanting sexual union form the 'leaping hare' mark.
(17–20)

The 'lotus leaf' mark is made in that shape on the front of

the breast or around the hips. The man going on a long journey should leave three or four 'line' marks close to each other on the woman's thighs or the front of her breasts for remembrance. These are the ways of using fingernails.
(21–22)

Thoughts on Scratching

Marks can also be made in other shapes. There is no end to options or to ingenuity in their usage. Passion is the inspiration and practice can take one anywhere. As such, say the teachers, no one can catalogue all the forms of scratching.
(23–24)

According to Vatsyayana, variety is a need even in passion. It generates mutual desires. Its skilful use makes elite courtesans and their lovers sought after by each other. It is no less a requirement in love than it is even in sciences such as archery and in other martial arts. But it should not be practised on the wives of others, though scratch marks may be made on the concealed parts of their bodies, specially as mementoes to enhance their love.
(25–26)

> When a woman sees nail marks
> made upon her secret places,
> her love renews its tenderness
> though abandoned long ago.
> When passion has been long forsaken
> love would also disappear
> unless there were marks of nails,
> reminders of a store of bliss.

Respect for her, desire too,
rise even in a stranger who
sees a young woman from afar,
her breasts bearing marks of nails.
And the minds of women too,
stolid even though they be,
are often set to take a toss
on seeing nail marks on a man.
So, for the stoking-up of passion
there is nothing keener than
the results to be got
from the use of nails and teeth.
(27–31)

CHAPTER FIVE:

Biting

The Places

The areas for biting with the teeth are the same as those for kissing, except for the upper lip, the inside of the mouth and the eyes.
(1)

Care of the Teeth

Good teeth are even, glossy and proportionate in size. They have sharp edges with no chips, and can be coloured. Those of

bad quality are blunt, out of line, rough, uneven, soft, broad and with spaces between them.
(2–3)

Kinds of Bite

There are different kinds of bite: the 'hidden', the 'swollen', the 'spot', the 'garland of spots', the 'coral and gem', the 'garland of gems', the 'piece of cloud' and the 'boar's bite'.
(4)

The 'hidden' bite is one that leaves just a hint of colour, not too red. And when it is done with pressure, it is called the 'swollen'. Both of these, applied to the middle of the lower lip, form the 'spot'.
(5–7)

The 'swollen' and the 'coral and gem' bites can be done on the cheek. It may be added that marks made by the nails and the teeth, as also by an earring and a kiss, are considered adornments of the left cheek.
(8–9)

The 'coral and gem' bite consists of pressing repeatedly with both the teeth as well as the lips, and several of these are called the 'garland of gems'. The 'spot' is made by using two teeth like a pair of tweezers on a small patch of skin, with many of these together forming a 'garland of spots'. Both garlands can be applied to the neck, the armpit and at the place where the thighs join the body. The 'garland of spots' is also made on the forehead and the thighs.
(10–15)

The 'piece of cloud' is made on the top of the breast, like a circle with uneven points. Several long lines of teeth marks on

the breast, made close to each other so that there is redness in-between, are known as the 'boar's bite'. These two are only for couples whose sexual impulse is intense.
(16–18)

Such are the forms of biting. Nail and bite marks made on floral decorations for the forehead and the ears, and on flower bouquets, betel and cinnamon bay leaves intended for a woman are also signs of a man's advances.
(19)

Regional Practices*

A woman should be treated in keeping with the practices of the land she comes from.
(20)

The women of Madhya Desha are generally noble and pure in conduct. They dislike kissing, scratching and biting. So do the women of Bahlika and Avanti, though they have expectations of variety in sex.
(21–23)

The ladies of Malava and Abhira give importance to hugging and kissing, also scratching, biting and sucking. They can be brought to a climax with slaps, but one must not wound them. The women of the land between the Indus and the other five rivers like oral sex.
(24–25)

Those of Aparanta and Lata have intense sexual impulses and moan softly. Those of Kosala and the kingdom of women harbour extremely fierce sexual impulses. They like to be hit hard and prefer the use of sex tools.
(26–27)

The Andhra women love sex and are gentle by nature, but have dirty tastes and coarse habits. The women of Maharashtra like to use all the sixty-four arts. They also enjoy rough and obscene talk and are quick to take the initiative in bed. The women of the City are the same, but they reveal this only in private.
(28–30)

Dravidian women moisten very slowly when stimulated during sex. The women of Vanavasa have a moderate sexual impulse. They can tolerate everything, but they hide their bodies and laugh at those of others. They also shun men who are low, vulgar and rough. The women of Gauda are loving, soft-spoken and have delicate limbs.
(31–33)

Suvarnanabha says that the individual's nature is more important than the regional practice, which matters less. It should also be understood that practices, costumes and pastimes follow each other from country to country over time.
(34–35)

Among the embraces and other things here described, those which increase passion should be used first and those which provide variety only later.
(36)

Retaliation

> Though warded off, if still the man
> wounds her body, and she cannot
> bear it – then retaliate
> and do it to him twice as hard.
> (37)

Countering the 'spot' with a 'garland',
and the 'garland' with a 'piece of cloud',
she responds with a battle,
pretending to be angry.
She grabs his hair and, raising
his mouth, kisses it long and hard,
embracing and biting him
everywhere like one drunk with love.
(39–40)
And when she sees him in a crowd,
even in daytime, displaying
the marks she has herself created,
she laughs unnoticed by the others
and reveals, as if with scorn,
the marks made on her own body,
while seeming to rebuke the man
with her face all screwed up.
(41–42)
Modest, caring for each other,
when a couple thus carry on,
their mutual love will never fade
even in a hundred years.
(43)

CHAPTER SIX:

Methods of Intercourse

A General Consideration

In the high union, where the male organ is larger in proportion to the female, a doe woman couples with a man by stretching out her pelvic area at the time of passion. In the low union, where she is larger, an elephant woman contracts herself. In an equal coupling the woman keeps her back straight. What has been said of the other two cases also applies to the mare woman. (1–4)

Methods described by Babhravya

The woman receives a man within her pelvic opening. Artificial means can also be used, particularly in the low union. (5–6)

The doe woman generally has three possibilities: the 'dilation', the 'yawn' and that named 'Indrani'. In the first, her head is kept low and the pelvis raised, though there must be room for the man to move back. The second requires her thighs to be lifted and spread wide apart to receive the man. In the third she puts her thighs around the man's sides and draws her knees back towards her own sides. This method needs practice but can be used even in the highest union. (7–12)

In the low union, where the woman is larger than the man, she receives him by cupping him inside her. This can be done even in the lowest union by an elephant woman. There are four methods: the 'box', the 'squeeze', the 'encirclement' and 'like a mare'. In the first, both man and woman stretch out their legs straight and keep them together. Depending on how they proceed, there are two variants: 'box' lying on the side and 'box' lying supine. While lying on their sides, the man should have the woman lie on his left, which is the general practice. (13–18)

For the man to press the woman's two thighs together tightly while cupped inside her is the 'squeeze' method, and if she then crosses her thighs, it is the 'encirclement'. To grasp him inside her as hard as a mare does a stallion is called 'like a mare'. It requires practice and is generally used by the women of Andhra. Such are the methods of intercourse described by the followers of Babhravya. (19–22)

Methods described by Suvarnanabha

According to Suvarnanabha, when the woman raises both her thighs to let the man enter, it is the 'bending' method, and when the man holds her legs up for this, it is the 'yawning'. When she draws up her legs beneath him, it is the 'pressing hard' and when only one of her legs is thus drawn up, it is the 'half-pressing'. When she stretches out one foot, placing it on the man's shoulder, and alternates this position with the other foot as they do this repeatedly, it is called 'splitting the bamboo'. (23–28)

When the woman raises one leg above her head while the other is stretched out, it is the 'impalement on a spear'. This method requires practice. In the 'crab', she draws up both her feet towards

the region of her navel, and in the 'pressing' method she raises and crosses her thighs. To separate her knees and cross her legs is the 'lotus position'. In the 'rotation' the man turns around after entering her while she embraces his back. This too needs practice.
(29–33)

Suvarnanabha says that various methods can also be practised while standing, sitting or lying down in water, as it makes them easier. This may be so, according to Vatsyayana, but it is not proper as learned people have proscribed it.
(34–35)

Unusual Sex*

Now some unusual methods of intercourse. Young couples do it standing up, leaning against each other's bodies, against a wall or a pillar. This is the 'stand-up' union.
(36–37)

He leans against a wall. She sits astride the net made by his clasped hands, her arms around his neck and her thighs encircling his hips, moving herself back and forth with her feet shifting on the wall. This is the 'suspended' union.
(38)

She goes down on the ground on all fours and he mounts her like a bull. This is the 'cow' union. In it he does on her back all that he would have done on her chest. This union is also like those of the dog, the stag and the billy-goat; the donkey's assault and the tom-cat's frolic; the tiger's spring and the elephant's crush; the pounding of the boar and the mounting of the stallion. In each of these he can consider doing whatever is special and peculiar to these animals.
(39–41)

Intercourse with two women who have good feelings for each other is known as the 'combination'. The same with many women is called the 'herd of cows'. It can be a dalliance in water or like those of goats and deer, whose actions can be imitated. (42–44)

In the kingdom of women, in regions with villages of women and in Bahlika, many young men have sex with one woman, as if they form her seraglio. They please her one by one or together, depending on her wish and what is doable. One holds and another services her: one between the legs, another in the mouth and yet another around the middle. They do this by turns and also in unison. Such group sex is also known among courtesans and the women of royal harems. (45–48)

The people of the south also have what is called nether sex, even in the anus. These are the unusual methods of sex. We will speak about the male approach in the chapter on reversing roles. There are two verses explaining the foregoing: (49–50)

> A man who knows the minds of women
> may amplify love's methods by
> the modes and by the manners of
> animals, wild beasts and birds.
> (51)

> For, when her feelings are excited
> in keeping with her temperament
> and the practice of her land,
> it inspires in a woman
> love, passion and great respect.
> (52)

CHAPTER SEVEN:
Hitting and Moaning

Kinds of Blow

It is said that, as love can also be disputatious and contrary, there is an aspect of conflict to sexual intercourse. Thus hitting is a part of it. The places for this are the two shoulders, the head, between the breasts, on the back, the pelvis and the sides. There are four ways of hitting: with the back of the hand, the hollowed hand, the fist and the flat of the palm.
(1–3)

Kinds of Moan*

Blows lead to moans expressive of pain. Of these there are several types, with eight kinds of sounds: the whimper, the groan, the babble, the wail, the sigh, the shriek, the sob and words with a meaning, such as 'Mother!' 'Stop!' 'Let go!' or 'Enough!' Cries like those of doves, cuckoos, green pigeons, parrots, bees, moorhens, geese, ducks and quails are important options for use in moaning.
(4–8)

Hitting during Sex

While she sits in his lap, the man strikes the woman on her back with his fist and, as if unable to bear this, she groans, wails and babbles, hitting him in return.
(9–10)

When he is inside her, he strikes her between the breasts with the back of his hand, at first gently, and then faster as her passion mounts, until it consummates. At the same time she moans continually in different ways, though there is no rule or order in whimpers and the other sounds.
(11–13)

If she sobs and protests, he strikes her on the head with his hand hollowed and the fingers slightly curled and, choking back her babbling and sobbing within her mouth, she sighs and weeps when intercourse ends.
(14–16)

The shriek is a sound like a bamboo splitting and the sob like a berry dropping into water. While moaning she should also always respond in kind when kisses and other things are forced upon her.
(17–19)

Driven by passion, when he hits her repeatedly she should mix words like 'Stop!' 'Let go!' 'Mother!' with sounds of laboured sighs, wails and groans. As passion nears its peak he may beat her faster on the pelvis and the sides until the climax. At this she should babble fast like a quail or a goose. Such are the ways of hitting and groaning. There are two verses about this:
(20–21)

> Ferocity and roughness are
> in man's nature, it is said;
> for woman it is lack of power,
> suffering and giving up,
> and a sense of weakness.
> These may sometime get reversed
> by passion and the methods used,

but not for long, as in the end
their natural state returns.
(22–23)

Southern Practices

The southern people hit in four other ways: the 'wedge' on the
chest, the 'scissors' on the head, the 'stabber' on the cheeks and
the 'pincer' on the breasts and the sides. Together with those
already described, this makes for eight methods of hitting.
Marks of the 'wedge' and similar blows can be seen on the
chests of young southern women. These are local practices.
(24)

According to Vatsyayana these practices are hurtful, barbaric
and unworthy of respect. The local customs of one place should
not be applied in another and dangerous methods should in any
case be avoided. The Chola king killed the courtesan Chitrasena
by using the 'wedge' blow in their sexual intercourse. Shatava-
hana Shatakarni of Kuntala did the same to his chief queen
Malayavati with the 'scissors', and Naradeva of the deformed
hand blinded a dancing girl in one eye by misusing the 'stabber'.
(25–30)

Conclusion

There are some verses on this:

> There is no counting of the ways
> nor adherence to the rules:
> once the act of love begins,

its only source is passion.
The fancies and emotions
which spring up within a moment
in intercourse can never be,
even in dreams, imagined.
Just as a galloping horse,
blind to all else by its pace,
is heedless of ditch, post or trench
which may be there within its path,
so two lovers blind with passion
in the fray of intercourse
let loose their most intense impulses
and pay no heed to any danger.
(31–33)

Therefore, having understood
a young woman's sex impulse,
its tenderness, ferocity,
her staying power and his own,
a man learned in this science
should then act accordingly.
For, these erotic methods
are not for using at all times
nor on all women:
a decision on their usage
should depend upon the place,
the region and the time.
(34–35)

CHAPTER EIGHT:

Reversing Roles

The Occasions and the Way

If her lover is exhausted with the constant repetition of his movement but his passion is not yet satisfied, the woman may, with his consent, push him down under her and help by herself acting out the man's role. She may also do this because of her own wish for a change or to satisfy the man's curiosity. (1–3)

She should move to the top with his organ still inside her, and place him below. In this way intercourse can continue without interruption of erotic feelings. This is one option. The other is to start all over again after she comes on top. (4–5)

Thereafter she may reciprocate all the actions her lover had earlier exhibited. Breathing hard and laughing, she presses hard on his chest with her breasts as she tries again and again to join her mouth to his, bending her head and scattering the flowers in her hair. 'You got me down!' she says with a laugh as she threatens and beats him, 'I do the same to you in return!' Then she may show signs of embarrassment, fatigue and a wish to stop, having proceeded exactly as does a man. (6)

The Male Approach*

We now speak of the male approach. When the woman is on the bed, the man as it were distracts her mind with talk and

loosens the knot of her skirt. If she argues, he overwhelms her with kisses on her cheeks.
(7–8)

His penis having become hard, he caresses her here and there: between her thighs, which she would have closed together tightly if it is their first time or she is a virgin girl, on her breasts, which she would have covered with her hands, and on her armpits, shoulders and neck.
(9–12)

With an experienced woman he does whatever suits them both and the occasion. He may pull back her hair mercilessly and grasp her chin with his fingers in order to kiss her.
(13)

An embarrassed woman will close her eyes, specially in a first encounter and if she is a virgin. So the man should observe her closely and consider what will please her during their sexual union. To whichever part of her body she turns her gaze when he is moving inside her, he should press her there. This is the secret of young women's arousal according to Suvarnanabha.
(14–16)

The signs of a woman nearing climax are that her limbs go limp, her eyes close, her bashfulness disappears and she takes the man deeper inside her. On the other hand, if he has already finished, she flings her hands, breaks into a sweat, bites, kicks and will not let him get up, acting even more like a man. So, before inserting his penis the man should first put his hand inside her, like an elephant's trunk, and excite her vagina till it becomes moist and soft. Only then should he enter her.
(17–19)

Types of Insertion

The man's actions after entering the woman are described as: moving, churning, piercing, grinding, pressing, striking, the boar's stroke, the bull's stroke, the sparrow's frolic and the box. (20)

The first is regular, straight intercourse. In the churning he rotates his penis with his hand in all directions inside her. In the piercing he pushes her pelvis down and thrusts into her from above. Reverse of this is the grinding, in which he raises her pelvis and thrusts violently from below. (21–24)

To stab into her with the penis and stay there long, putting pressure inside, is the pressing. And when he pulls himself out quite far and then brings his pelvis down hard upon the woman, it is known as the striking. The boar's thrust is to scrape inside her many times but only on one side. To do it alternately on both sides is the bull's thrust. (25–28)

Without pulling out after having joined with the woman, to thrust into her successively, two, three or four times is the sparrow's frolic. And the box, which has already been described, is employed as passion fades. The woman's nature should be taken into account in using any of these methods. (29–31)

Variations

There are three more methods when the roles are reversed and the woman acts the man: the 'pincer', the 'spinning top' and the 'swing'. (32)

In the first, she draws his penis inside her like a mare, squeezing and pressing it there for a long time. In the second, she turns like a wheel with the penis inside her. This needs practice, and the man should then thrust his own pelvis upwards. And in the third, she swings her pelvis in all directions.
(33–36)

With the man still inside her, she can also rest, laying her forehead against his. And, after she has rested, the man can again come on top of her. Such is the reversal of roles. There are some verses about it:
(37–38)

Though a woman keeps concealed
her feelings, hides her actions too,
all emotion is laid bare
when passion gets her on the top.
(39)

How is the woman's disposition,
and for sex her eagerness:
all of this a man may see
from the way she moves up there.
(40)

A woman, though, should not be put
to act the man in roles reversed,
if she is pregnant or in period,
or recently has given birth,
or is a 'doe' or very fat.
(41)

CHAPTER NINE:

Oral Sex

The Third Nature: Feminine

The third nature is of two kinds, feminine and masculine. That of the feminine kind imitates women in appearance and talk, gestures and emotions, softness and timidity, whimsicality, impatience and bashfulness. What is done in the pubes of a woman is done in her mouth. This is known as oral sex. She derives her erotic satisfaction as well as livelihood from it, living the life of a courtesan. Such is the feminine type. (1–5)

The Third Nature: Masculine

The masculine type must hide her desire, but wants a man. She works as a masseur to make a living. In the course of massage, as if rubbing a man's limbs, she clasps both his thighs and, becoming more familiar, touches him in the groin and the pelvis. Getting his penis to harden, she takes it in her fist, moving it about as she laughs and teases him for his haste. If the man does not urge her to proceed further even after he has shown signs of arousal, she takes the initiative herself. But if he urges her on, she argues and continues only on persuasion. (6–11)

Oral Sex

The act consists of eight elements: the 'nominal', the 'biting the sides', the 'outer pincer', the 'inner pincer', the 'kiss', the 'lick', the 'sucking the mango' and the 'swallowing'. These should be done one by one, and after each she should exhibit a wish to stop. As for the man, on the conclusion of one he should ask for the next, and when that too is done, for the one after that.
(12–15)

She takes the penis in her hand and, placing it on her lips, puts it in her mouth which she moves back and forth. This is the 'nominal'. Then, covering its forepart with her hand, she nibbles the sides with her lips without biting, and consoles him, saying 'Only so much!' This is 'biting the sides'.
(16–17)

Urged by the man to continue, she closes her lips around the forepart, squeezing and kissing it as if to draw it out. This is the 'outer pincer'. On his further insistence, she takes it in a little deeper and spits it out after a squeeze with her lips. This is the 'inner pincer'.
(18–19)

In the 'kiss' she holds the penis in her hand and takes it in as if it were his lip. Then, rubbing it all over with the tip of her tongue, she probes its front: that is the 'lick'.
(20–21)

After that, taking half the penis in as passion mounts, she squeezes it mercilessly and repeatedly before releasing it: that is called 'sucking the mango'. And to swallow and squeeze till the very end: that is the 'swallowing', which should only be done if the man desires it. Slaps and sighs can also be used as required. Such is oral sex. Women, too, engage in it: wanton

and promiscuous women, servant maids and those who work as masseuses.
(22–25)

Opinions and Practices

According to learned teachers, oral sex should not be practised. It is against convention and civilized behaviour. And, if the man subsequently has contact with that woman's mouth, he may himself find it distasteful.
(26)

According to Vatsyayana, however, it is not a flaw in a man who goes to a courtesan, even though it is avoidable elsewhere. Thus, eastern men do not have intercourse with women who practise oral sex. The men of Ahichhatra do not generally sleep with courtesans, and even when they do they avoid their mouths. And while the men of Saketa sleep with them without any inhibition, the gentlemen of the City do not themselves engage in oral sex. Those of Surasena, however, do everything without any hesitation.
(27–32)

It is said: Who can have faith in the character and purity of women, in their behaviour and action, their words and beliefs? But they can not be rejected as their uncleanliness comes from nature itself. So, their purity should be determined in accordance with the scriptures. And these have said:

> The calf is pure at milking time,
> the dog when it has caught a deer,
> the bird while pecking at fruit which falls,
> and a woman's mouth when making love.

As there is a discrepancy between learned opinion and scriptural pronouncement, one should act according to the occasion, the local practice and one's own inclination and belief. This is the view of Vatsyayana.
(33–34)

There are some verses on this subject:

> Even young men and servants
> with well-polished earrings
> perform oral sex,
> but only with certain men.
> Some city men too,
> who are mutually caring
> and trustful as well,
> do this with each other.
> (35–36)

> Men indeed perform this act
> on women also: its method then,
> it should be known,
> is like a kiss upon the mouth.
> Their bodies inverted mutually,
> one's head towards the other's feet,
> to have each other, both together:
> such coupling of a man and woman
> is known as making love like crows.
> (37–38)

> Thus is it that harlots give up
> men of merit, skilful, liberal,
> and get attached instead to villains,
> servants, elephant grooms and suchlike.

But learned brahmins, or ministers
responsible for state affairs,
or those relied on for their knowledge,
should not engage in oral sex.
(39–40)

That there are scriptural rules about it
cannot sanction doing it,
for scriptures deal with everything
but use depends upon each case.
Medical texts say even dog's meat,
cooked, will enhance virility.
Should it therefore be consumed
by people with intelligence?
(41–42)

Indeed there are people
and places and times
where and when such practices
are not without use.
So, having considered
the place, the time, the usage,
the scriptures and also oneself,
one may or not engage in it.
As the mind is always fickle
and the motive is a secret,
none can claim to know
when and where and who will do it.
(43–45)

CHAPTER TEN:

Before and After

At the Start

A civilized man receives a woman with his friends in an inner
room meant for pleasure. The room would have been decorated with flowers and perfumed with incense by servants. The
woman would have bathed, made up and had some wine in
proper measure. He urges her gently to have some more.
(1)

He sits on her right. Touching her hair, the fringe of her garment and her skirt-knot with his hand, he embraces her softly
with his left arm to prepare for love-making.

> In joking and loving words,
> they recall their past encounters,
> talking with some half-said hints
> about secret and naughty things.

There may be singing and instrumental music, with or without dancing. They may talk about the fine arts and she may be
persuaded to have another drink.
(2–4)

Once her feelings are aroused, the other people are sent away
with gifts of flowers, scented balm and betel leaf. And when they
are alone he stimulates her further with embraces and the other
means. He then proceeds to loosen her skirt-knot and do the other
things already described. This is the prelude to sexual union.
(5)

At the End

At the end of intercourse, their passion spent, the couple may feel bashful and go separately to the bathroom without looking at each other, almost as if they are unacquainted. No more embarrassed on return, they sit in a suitable place and partake of betel leaf. He should then himself apply fresh sandalwood or another pomade to her limbs.
(6)

Embracing her with his left arm, he reassures her and offers her a drink from a wineglass held in his hand. Or they both drink water and have some snacks according to their choice: fresh juice and meat broth, sour porridge and bite-size bits of roast meat, beverages and mangoes, dried meat, citron and tamarind fruit with sugar, and others in keeping with local preferences. He tastes each before he offers them to her, saying 'This one is sweet', or 'Very delicate'. Or they go on the roof to enjoy the moonlight, and have a pleasant conversation. She reclines in his arms, gazing at the moon, and he points out the constellations. They look at Arundhati the morning star, Dhruva the pole star and Saptarshimala, the chain of the seven sages, which is the great bear. Such is the culmination of their union.
(7–9)

Reviving Passion

It is said:

> Even at its ending, pleasure
> still nurtured with caring acts

and words exchanged in confidence,
causes a supreme delight.
Responding to each other's feelings
which inspire mutual pleasure –
one moment a show of anger,
in the next a loving gaze –
they play at ring around the roses,
they sing, they dance the Lata way,
their eyes rolling, moist with passion,
they stare at the orb of the moon.
Talking of old times,
the wishes they both had
at their very first meeting
and the sadness and pain
when they were parted,
and after this ardent
embraces and kisses.
With such exchanges
passion increases.
(10–13)

Kinds of Sex*

The kinds of sex are: passionate or with a cultivated passion, with a passion artificial or transferred, with a low woman, with a base person and uninhibited sex.
(14)

Passionate sex is that in which the feelings of a couple for each other grow from their first meeting and they make efforts to get together again or meet on return from a long journey or after a separation caused by a quarrel. It lasts as long as they

wish, till the climax. However, when they begin with a desire still tepid and it then grows into a pleasurable feeling, that is called cultivated passion. It can be enhanced with stimulation by any of the sixty-four methods the couple prefer.
(15–18)

Intercourse with artificial passion is that which takes place for some particular purpose or when the couple are attracted elsewhere. In it one should apply the gamut of techniques as prescribed. And when, from the beginning of intercourse to its climax, the man proceeds with his thoughts on another woman dear to his heart, that is sex with transferred passion.
(19–21)

Sex with a low woman is that done up to the climax with an inferior water-carrier or servant girl. In it there is no need for preliminaries. Similar is sex with a base person, when a courtesan has it with some rustic to reach her own climax, or a gentleman with women from villages, pasture lands and forest regions. Uninhibited sex takes place between couples who are suited to each other and have mutual trust. Such are the kinds of sex.
(22 –26)

The Quarrel in Love*

In the course of love-making a woman may not be able to endure her lover remembering his co-wife, calling her by that woman's name or talking about her. Nor will she tolerate his lying. Then there is a mighty quarrel: weeping, pulling of hair, hitting, falling off the seat or from the bed to the floor, tearing off garlands and jewellery and lying down on the ground.
(27–28)

Keeping his calm, the lover conciliates her. He tries to please

her with sweet words and by falling at her feet, to take her back to bed. But her anger increases as she answers him back. Grabbing his hair, she pulls him up, kicks him a couple of times on his arms or his head, his chest or his back and goes to the door, where she sits and sheds copious tears.
(29–30)

Even if she is very angry, according to Dattaka she should not go out of the door as that would be a mistake. Properly conciliated, she should turn gracious at the door itself. But even though pleased and ready to renew love-making, she should say something sarcastic, as if to needle her lover when he embraces her.
(31)

Her lover's approach should be similar when she is in her own house and they have quarrelled for some reason. He sends his companions, hangers-on and jesters to her house. Conciliated by them and her anger pacified, she should return with them to her lover's house and spend the night there. This concludes the quarrel of lovers.
(32–33)

The Sixty-four Methods

Here are some concluding verses:

> Such are they, the four and sixty
> that Babhravya did speak about,
> that a lover using them will have
> success with his chosen woman.
> Even though a man may discourse
> on other subjects and their rules,

if of the sixty-four devoid,
his words in learned assemblies
will not be much respected.
And, though lacking other knowledge,
one illumined with this learning
will the leading light become
in gatherings of men and women.
For, who will not respect this pleasant
science, honoured by the learned,
and, more so, even by the wicked,
and by guilds of courtesans?
Teachers, even scriptures, call it
joyous, bringer of good fortune,
success and of luck in love,
and one dear to women.
An expert in the sixty-four
is with great respect regarded
by virgin girls and others' wives,
and by elite courtesans.
(34–39)

BOOK THREE

The Maiden

CHAPTER ONE:

Arranging a Marriage

The Objective

A woman of the same caste who has not been with another man before, when taken in marriage lawfully, helps in a man's pursuit of Dharma and Artha and provides him with progeny, connections, more friends and straightforward sexual pleasure. A wise man should therefore cultivate a virgin girl with a good background and with both her parents living. At least three years younger than himself, she is from a respectable, wealthy and well-connected family, dear to her relations and well integrated with them. Her mother's and her father's kin are both numerous. She has good looks, a nice disposition and lucky signs on her body. Her teeth and nails, ears and eyes, hair and breasts are unspoilt and neither too small nor too big. Also, she should not be sickly by nature.
(1–2)

Ghotakamukha adds that the girl chosen should be one in taking whom a man will consider himself fulfilled and not be criticized by his peers.
(3)

How to Proceed

A man's parents and relations try to ask for the girl's hand. So too do friends connected to both sides who could act as go-betweens. To strengthen their case they might dwell on the merits of the man's family and his personality, comparing them with the obvious and probable deficiencies of other suitors. In particular they point out the man's present and future qualities which the girl's mother may find congenial. One goes disguised as a soothsayer and predicts the man's good fortune and acquisition of wealth by referring to omens, signs and the strength of his planetary positions in the zodiac. Others make the girl's mother anxious by suggesting that the man may find another, even better girl.

(4–7)

Girls to Avoid

Signs, omens and sounds indicative of good fortune should be followed in choosing a girl, and not just people's preference, says Ghotakamukha. A girl who is asleep, weeping or absent is not to be considered for marriage. Nor one with an inauspicious name, one kept hidden or one already betrothed. Nor a girl with red hair, with white spots on her body, bull-like, stooping, hideous or bald. Nor one whose purity has been polluted, who is promiscuous, menstruating or pregnant. Nor a childhood friend like one's own younger sister or one who perspires too much.

> Neither should one marry
> women with despised names
> of constellations, rivers, trees,
> or ones which end in syllables beginning
> with the letters 'l' and 'r'.

According to one opinion, the girl who can catch a man's eye and capture his heart will also bring him good fortune. One should not consider any other.
(8–13)

Making the Alliance

A girl ripe for marriage should be attired in all her finery. Always well dressed, she moves about with her girl friends in the afternoon. Attempts are made to display her thus at public gatherings such as sacrifices, weddings and festivals, just like a piece of merchandise.
(14)

Nice-looking, well-spoken suitors should be received with all civilities. The girl is adorned and shown to them under some pretext, and a time frame set for checking fateful signs till a decision is taken on the marriage. Should the girl's side propose the ceremonial bath and so forth, the suitor's side need not agree to have it on the same day, saying 'This is for the future'. Then the girl should be taken in marriage according to the scriptures with the *Brahma*, *Prajapatya*, *Arsha* or *Daiva* rites in keeping with the local practice. This concludes the arrangement of a marriage.
(15–19)

A Decisive Point*

There are some verses on this:

> Marriages, like making friends,
> and games with others like verse-capping,

should always only be with equals;
never with the people who
are higher than one or below.
The alliance in which a man
takes a girl, but then must live
like a serf is called 'the high'
and the wise avoid it.
And one in which he moves about
like the master, waited on
by his in-laws and their kin
is the worthless 'low' alliance,
condemned by all good people.
The alliance most recommended
is that in which the two accord
precedence to one another –
a pleasure giving both of them
the taste of mutual happiness.
(20–23)

Having made a 'high' alliance,
one must to all the kin bow down:
still, never make the 'low' alliance
which good people censure.
(24)

CHAPTER TWO:

Winning the Girl's Trust

The First Three Nights

After their marriage, for the first three nights a couple should sleep on the floor and observe celibacy. Pungent and salty food is abjured. For a week they have ceremonial baths accompanied by music, dress up and eat together, attend shows and visit relatives. This is done by all the classes.
(1)

During this period, when they are alone at night, the man should make gentle advances to the girl. For, as pointed out by the followers of Babhravya, if she sees him act a silent statue for three nights, she may think he is of the third nature and despise him. So he should make advances and assure her, according to Vatsyayana. But he should not transgress the bounds of celibacy, nor should he do anything to coerce her.
(3-5)

Winning Trust Gently

Girls are like flowers and need to be approached with a certain delicacy. If the approach is violent before gaining their trust, they could be turned off sex altogether. So it must be gentle, even if contrived, and the man should feel his way along.
(6-7)

So he should embrace her in a way that pleases her, but not for too long, and only with the upper half of his body which

she can endure. A mature young woman he already knows well can be embraced with the lamp light still on, but if she is a girl he does not know at all, he should approach her in the dark.
(8–10)

Moves towards Sex

Once she accepts his embraces, he offers her a betel leaf with his mouth. Should she be reluctant, he persuades her with words of assurance, oaths, counter-proposals or even by falling at her feet. The last a girl will generally not ignore even if she is embarrassed or very angry. And then, while putting the betel leaf in her mouth, he kisses her softly, without a sound.
(11–12)

This achieved, he gets her to talk. Pretending he does not know something, he asks whatever can be answered in a few words, just to listen to her voice. If she does not reply, he asks again, always reassuringly and never by agitating her. If she still does not speak, he should persist, for, as Ghotakamukha states, all girls comprehend what men say though they may not utter a word, even as small talk.
(13–17)

Unlike what happens in a quarrel, when the man persists she will answer by nodding or shaking her head. Thus, pressed for long with 'Do you want me?' or 'Don't you want me?', 'Do you like me?' or 'You don't like me?', she replies with a shake or a nod. If tricked into doing so, she may argue about it.
(18–19)

If they already know each other, the man can begin their conversation with the intermediary of a woman friend trusted

by both and well inclined towards him. Then the girl lowers her gaze and smiles. If the friend talks too much she chides and argues with her. 'She said this,' the friend may joke, even when the girl has said nothing. And when the man follows up and asks for an answer, she remains silent. 'I am not saying any such thing,' she replies at last in indistinct and unclear words when the man persists, and smiles as she casts a sidelong glance at him. This is how he gets her to talk.
(20–21)

When she has thus got to know him, and they are alone, she puts near him without a word the betel leaf, the pomade and the garland he asked for. Or she ties them to his upper garment. While she is thus occupied he brushes her on the nipples with the 'mixed' touch. If she protests, he says: 'You embrace me too. Then I will not do this,' and then embraces her. Stretching his hand down to her navel, he first withdraws it and, by degrees getting her on his lap, goes further and further. If she resists he makes a mock threat. 'I will definitely make bite marks on your lower lip and scratch marks on your breast. Then, doing the same to myself, I will tell your girl friends that you made them. What will you say then?' Thus does he beguile her, bit by bit, like children are cajoled with threats and assurances.
(22–24)

On the second and the third nights, when she is a little more assured, he works on her with his hands, and kisses her all over. Placing his hand on her thighs, he caresses them, moving gradually even to where they join her body. If she restrains him, he confuses her by saying 'What's wrong in this?' and goes slow till he succeeds and touches her secret place. Then he loosens her girdle, unties the skirt-knot, turns up the garment and resumes caressing her groins, all under various pretexts. Finally

he penetrates and pleasures her. But the vow of celibacy for the first three nights should not be broken before its time.
(25–28)

Thereafter he teaches her in the ways of love, demonstrates his own love for her and tells her about his ambitions in the past. Promising to live in the way she wants, he also dispels her anxiety about co-wives. And, though she is no longer a virgin, he continues to make advances gradually over the course of time without agitating her. This concludes the winning of a girl's trust.
(29)

Merits of the Gradual Approach

Here are some verses on this:

> The man who follows a maiden's mind
> can win it over in this way
> by stratagems which make her love
> and begin to trust him.
> Winning a girl cannot be done
> just by falling in line with her,
> nor by going against her wishes:
> one should steer a middle course.
> The man who can inspire
> love for himself in a girl,
> by increasing her self-respect
> and winning her confidence
> will be very dear to her.
> But one who will neglect a girl,
> considering her to be too shy –

she despises as a beast
who cannot comprehend her.
Or, unmindful of her feelings,
one who forces himself on a girl,
will plunge her forthwith in a state
of fear, alarm, regret and hate.
Thus denied the pleasure of love,
and by regrets overcome,
she becomes a man-hater, or,
vengeful, turns to other men.
(30–35)

CHAPTER THREE:

Approaching a Maiden

Where to Begin

A man with no money even though meritorious, one of average merit but with a bad reputation, a next-door neighbour though rich, one dependent on his parents and brothers or one admitted into the house only because of his childlike disposition: such a man will not be able to marry a girl in the ways described earlier. He can, however, try to win one by cultivating her from her childhood.
(1–2)

Such a man in the south, a poor orphan living with the family of his mother's brother, can win over that uncle's daughter though she may be rich and unattainable or already betrothed to someone else. He can also try for another girl outside the

family. Such courting for the sake of Dharma is praiseworthy, according to Ghotakamukha, even with a young girl.
(3–5)

How to Proceed

In keeping with their familiarity and ages, he can go picking flowers with the girl, stringing them into garlands, playing house with dolls or preparing meals. He can also play with her and her trusted servants and maids at dice and board, betting with fists and shells, catching the middle finger, six pebbles and other local games she likes. With her girl friends they can play livelier games like hide and seek, starters, line of salt, hitting the wind, heaps of wheat, finger strikes and others of the region.
(6–8)

He thus gets to know and constantly pleases the girl friend whom she trusts. In particular he is attentive to the daughter of the girl's nurse. If she likes him, she will not come in his way, even if she knows his intentions, but will bring him together with the girl and also advise him unasked. And, even if unaware, she can publicize his merits out of love for him so as to attract the girl he wants to woo.
(9–11)

He finds out what interests the girl and arranges to provide it. Playthings she has never had before, which girls seldom know of, he gets her right away. He shows her balls with many stripes of variegated quickly changing colours, dolls of string and wood, horn and ivory, wax, dough or clay, and demonstrates utensils for cooking rice. He gives her presents, secretly where he can and openly those which are for public display: little coupling sheep made of wood; a pair of wooden figures,

man and woman, joined together; small temples of clay, split bamboo and wood for the families of gods; cages for parrots and cuckoos, mynahs and quails, cocks and partridges; water pots of various shapes; clockwork toys and lutes; cosmetics like lac, red and yellow arsenic, vermilion and collyrium, sandalwood and saffron; areca nuts and leaves in season. He tries to convince her that he is someone who can meet all her desires.
(12–16)

Making up a story, he asks to see her in private, and explains that his fear of elders was the reason for his secret gift, also that others may have wanted it. As her love grows and she evinces interest in more stories, he entertains her with suitable tales which will steal her heart away. If she delights in marvels, he performs magic tricks to astonish her; if she is curious about the fine arts, he demonstrates his skills in them; if fond of music, he amuses her with captivating songs. During her visits to the moonlight celebration for the eighth moon of autumn, other festivals, eclipses or homecomings, he presents her with different kinds of chaplets, ear decorations, indigo dyed cloth, rings and other ornaments, but not if he thinks this will cause any misunderstanding.
(17–20)

He explains to the daughter of the girl's nurse the sixty-four techniques of love used by a man, so that she knows that he is different from other men, and also becomes aware of his expertise in sexual enjoyment. He dresses well, makes sure that the girl notices him and gauges her feelings from her gestures and expressions. Young women first come to like a man whom they know and who is always around but, even so, generally do not take the initiative. So much for approaching girls.
(21–24)

The Girl's Responses*

Here we speak about the girl's gestures and expressions. She does not look at the man directly. Being noticed by him, she acts embarrassed. Under some pretext she exposes the attractive parts of her body. And she glances at him furtively, when he is distracted or at a distance.

(25–26)

Asked about something, she smiles and replies very softly in indistinct words with unclear meanings, her gaze downcast. She is pleased to be near him for a long time. If at a distance, she speaks with her attendants in a raised voice, hoping he will notice her, and does not leave that place. And she laughs at whatever she sees, talking about it to stay on there. She may kiss and hug a child in her arms, make a beauty spot on her maid and, with her attendants as the backdrop, put on all kinds of acts.

(27–28)

She confides in his friends, and respects and follows their advice. With his attendants she talks pleasantly and plays dice and other games. She also puts them to work like a superior and listens carefully to what they say to others about the man. Encouraged by her nurse's daughter, she goes to his house to play dice or have a chat with the daughter as a go-between. But she avoids coming before him unless she is all dressed up. If he asks for her ear ornament, ring or flower garland as a memento, she gravely takes it off and puts it in her girl friend's hand. What he gives her, she always wears. And if there is talk of other suitors, she becomes dejected and will have nothing to do with their supporters.

(29–30)

There are two verses here:

> Having seen her gestures and
> expressions imbued with feeling,
> the man should think of various ways
> for getting together with that girl.
> (31)

> A girl is won with children's games,
> a young woman with the arts,
> and one affectionate and mature
> by winning over those she trusts.
> (32)

CHAPTER FOUR:

The Man's Advances

The Man's Advances*

It is after seeing the girl's gestures and expressions that a man considers ways to make his advances. He can hold her hand with a meaningful look while contesting a point in the course of dice and other games. He can resort to the 'touch' and the other embraces already described. While cutting figures out of leaves he can hint at his own intentions by showing her, once in a while, a coupled pair among other images. While playing in the water he can dive down at a distance and come out near her after touching her. He can also express his special feelings with fresh tender leaves and suchlike, talk about his own unhappiness, but without self-pity, and tell her among other things of some emotional dream he has had.

(1–9)

He sits near her at shows and family gatherings, and touches her under some pretext. He presses her foot with his own placed upon it, touching each of her toes, one after the other, rubbing her toenails with his big toe. This achieved, he goes further, step by step, carrying on till she begins to tolerate it. While she is washing his feet he presses her fingers, using his toes as a pincer. After the ceremonial sipping of water, he sprinkles some on her, and, while giving her something or taking it from her, he makes a special mark upon it.

(10–18)

When they are sitting together alone in the dark, or reclining in the same area, he makes her feel comfortable and expresses his feelings without agitating her. 'I had something to tell you in private,' he says, alluding to some unexpressed emotion as described in the section on other men's wives. And once he knows her feelings for him, he gets her to visit his home on the pretext of obtaining his news as he is unwell. After her arrival he develops a headache and, taking her hand emotionally, places it upon his forehead and eyes. 'This act is therapeutic,' he says. 'It has to be performed by you. It can't be done by anyone except a virgin girl.' And when she is leaving he lets her go with many requests that she come again.

(19–25)

The foregoing method can be used for three evenings and nights. When she comes again he must talk with her at even greater length to ensure more frequent visits. Even if she comes with other women, he should continue to try winning her trust though he may not say anything in particular. For, as Ghotaka-

mukha observes, even when his feelings for a girl are far
advanced, a man cannot succeed without expressing them. But
his advances should be made only when he is sure that the girl
is well prepared to receive them. It is generally said that young
women are less timid in the evening, at night and in the dark.
They then become passionate, inclined to sex and will not
refuse a man. Therefore that is the time to have them.
(26–31)

Sometimes it is not possible for a man to make advances on
his own. He should then induce her girlfriend or her nurse's
daughter, who sympathize with him and know his intent, but
will be discreet, virtually to lead the girl into his arms so that he
may proceed as earlier described. Or he can have his own
housemaid installed as the girl's companion. Then he can make
his advances whenever other people are busy with sacrifices or
weddings, travelling or festivals, shows and other preoccupa-
tions, and the girl is alone. But he should first have judged her
feelings for him from her gestures and expressions. According
to Vatsyayana, once a woman has revealed her feelings she will
never turn away if approached at the right time and place. This
concludes the man's advances.
(32–35)

The Woman's Advances*

A girl of quality but from a modest background, well bred but
with no money, true to her family and class but an orphan, may
never be sought after by her peers for marriage. So, on coming
of age she should herself take the initiative in getting married.
(36)

She looks for a man of merit, able, handsome and known from childhood. Or one she thinks will want to marry of his own accord without consulting his parents because his flesh is weak. She should attract them with endearing ways and frequent meetings. Her mother, together with her girl friends and nurse's daughters, should also encourage her in this.
(37–39)

She meets the man in lonely places at odd hours, with flowers, perfumes or a betel leaf in hand. She displays her proficiency in the arts and skill in massaging and pressing the head. She talks to him about what he likes and conducts herself as described in the section on approaching a maiden. But she should not make overt advances to the man, even if she is so inclined. For a young woman doing this ruins her own future prospects, according to the teachers.
(40–41)

However, she goes along with the man's advances, not showing any excitement when embraced and accepting his gentler moves as if unaware of them. She lets herself be kissed only by force, and permits his touching her private parts with great difficulty when he begs her for this because of his erotic arousal. But she does not open herself up too much, even though entreated by him. For the time for that is still far off and uncertain.
(42–45)

It is only when she is sure that 'He loves me and will not leave me' that she lets the aroused man do away with her maidenhood. And when she has lost her virginity, she should make this known to those she trusts. Such are the woman's advances.
(46–47)

Winning the Maiden*

There are some verses here:

> A girl sought after
> should marry the man
> she thinks will give her
> a comfortable home,
> be someone compatible
> and in her control.
> (48)

> But, ignoring merit,
> appearance, propriety,
> out of greed for money
> when she looks for a husband,
> even one with other wives,
> she will not attract a man
> of quality, ability,
> wanting her strongly,
> seeking to get her,
> and one she could control.
> (49–50)

> Better a man controllable
> though he may be poor,
> able to support one
> though lacking other merits,
> than one endowed with them
> but a husband of many wives.
> For such wives of rich men

are often unrestrained,
go out for enjoyments
and have external comforts,
but no self-assurance.
(51–52)

A base man or a greybeard,
or one inclined to go abroad,
is not worth marrying
though he may make advances.
Nor one who propositions
just when it pleases him,
is an arrogant gambler
or has a wife and children.
(53–54)

If there are several suitors,
all with similar merits,
she should then select the one
with the most loving nature.
(55)

CHAPTER FIVE:
Other Types of Marriage

The Role of the Girl's Confidante

Often a man is unable to see a girl alone. He then cultivates her nurse's daughter with pleasing things and favours. She pretends that she does not know him at all, but gets the girl attracted to his qualities, emphasizing those she is bound to like. She also dwells on such defects of other suitors that are contrary to the girl's own wishes, and on her parents' greed, their inability to recognize merit and the casual attitude of her kinsfolk. She tells her about Shakuntala and others, even girls of her own class, who found husbands by their own efforts and lived with them happily. Giving examples from great families, where girls are oppressed by co-wives, hated, made miserable and abandoned, she talks of the man's love for her, of her future with him and of the faultless happiness of being his sole wife. (1–8)

The confidante carries out all the functions of a go-between. After the girl's feelings have been aroused she reasons with her to dispel any fear, anxiety or embarrassment she may still have. 'That man can just pretend to kidnap you,' she tells the girl, 'and others can then be pursuaded to accept it fully.' (9–11)

Formalizing the Marriage

Once the girl has agreed and comes to the man for the rendez-vous, he brings the sacred fire from the house of a priest who knows the Veda. Spreading the ritual *kusha* grass on the ground, he offers oblations into the fire in accordance with the scriptures and they walk round it three times in the act of marriage.

(12)

Her parents can then be informed. According to preceptors it is an established rule that a marriage witnessed by the sacred fire cannot be rescinded. And, after taking her maidenhead, the man gradually informs his own people. He so proceeds that the girl's kinsfolk will accept their marriage, both to avoid any ignominy for her family and out of fear of any reprisals. Thereafter he satisfies them with pleasing gifts and affectionate behaviour. Or, he proceeds with a *Gandharva* marriage or union of love.

(13–18)

If the girl is hesitant, he pursuades another woman of her family, who is intimate with her and already knows and likes him, to conduct her on some pretext to an accessible place where he brings the fire from the Veda-knowing priest's house and proceeds as earlier indicated.

(19–20)

If the girl is soon to be married elsewhere, he gets her mother to regret it by having her informed of the intended groom's defects. With her consent the girl is then brought at night to a neighbour's house where the man brings the fire from the priest and proceeds as earlier.

(21–22)

Or the girl may have a brother of the same age who is infatuated with some courtesan or another woman. The man cultivates him at length with pleasing gifts and help in his difficulties. Finally he tells him of his own desire. Young people are often prepared to stake even their lives for friends with

similar dispositions, vices and ages. Thus he has the girl's brother bring her for some other reason to an accessible place, and then proceeds as before.
(23–24)

Forcible Marriage

On festivals like that of the eighth night of the waxing moon, the girl is plied with some intoxicating drink by her nurse's daughter and taken on some personal pretext to a place accessible to the man. There he takes her maidenhead while she is drunk, and then proceeds as before.
(25)

After sending the nurse's daughter away, he takes the girl's maidenhead while she is alone, asleep and out of her senses, and then proceeds as before. Or, after coming to know that the girl is going to a park or another village, he goes with his servants and helpers, frightens away or kills her guards and abducts her. These are the other types of marriage.
(26–27)

Concluding Verses

For the maintenance of Dharma,
each preceding form of marriage
is better than that which comes next,
but if it is not possible, then
one may use the form which follows.
The fruit of every type of marriage
should be mutual love, and so

the good Gandharva is respected,
even though of middle rank.
It is indeed the best of all,
as giving pleasure, little trouble
and free of many rituals too,
its essence being mutual love.
(28–30)

BOOK FOUR

The Wife

CHAPTER ONE:

The Only Wife

Her Life and Conduct

The only wife has deep confidence in her husband and conforms to him as if he were a god. With his concurrence she takes the responsibility of the household upon herself. The house is kept clean and pleasing. The rooms are well swept and decorated with a variety of flowers, the floors polished and smooth. Sacrificial offerings at the shrine of the household deities are made thrice a day. Nothing is dearer to a householder's heart than this, according to Gonardiya. She pays due regard to the elders and the servants, to her husband's sisters and their spouses.
(1–5)

The grounds of the house are well weeded. There she plants beds of herbs and green vegetables, clumps of sugar cane, patches of cumin and mustard, anise and fennel and shrubs of cinnamon. In the park she prepares charming plots of muskrose and gooseberry, magnolia and jasmine, amaranth and verbena, rosebay, adam's apple and hibiscus, as well as other flowering plants like lemon grass, poppy and scurvy grass. A well, a tank or a pond is located in the middle of the park.
(6–8)

She does not associate with women who are mendicants, ascetics or nuns, wantons or cheats, soothsayers or sorcerers. In the preparation of food she bears in mind her husband's likes and dislikes, and what is good for him or not. Hearing his voice outside when he is coming home, she stands ready in the courtyard, calling out 'Anything needed?' and, brushing aside the servant maid, herself washes his feet.

(9–12)

She does not appear before her husband in private without any adornment. In all pleasures she follows his lead. If he spends money wrongly or excessively, she points this out only when they are alone. She goes to bed after he does, gets up before him and does not disturb him when he is asleep. The kitchen is kept well guarded and well lit. And when she goes out, to attend betrothals, weddings or sacrificial ceremonies, to meet her women friends or visit temples, it is with her husband's consent.

(13–18)

When a little offended at some misdoing of her husband, she does not speak to him too harshly. If she has to reproach him, she does it when they are alone or among close friends. But she never resorts to sorcery, for nothing destroys trust more than this, according to Gonardiya. She refrains from using bad language, looking daggers, speaking with her face turned away, standing in the doorway and staring, chatting with someone in the park and lingering in lonely places.

(19–22)

She takes care of bad odours – of perspiration and dirty teeth – for these can turn off a man. When going to make love, she adorns herself with jewellery, fragrant oils of various flowers, all kinds of powders and bright clothes. When going on a pleasure trip, she dresses in delicate, soft and light silks, with few ornaments and some scented but not too strong pomade, her hair done up with flowers both white and coloured.

(23–25)

The vows and fasts undertaken by her husband, she too observes herself. 'I cannot be prohibited in this,' she retorts if he stops her. When the time and the price are right she acquires household goods of clay, bamboo and wood, leather and iron. Also salt and oil, and hard-to-get fragrances, bitters and medicines which she keeps hidden in the house. She buys and sows at the appropriate time the seeds of all kinds of edible plants like radish, potato, beetroot, wormwood, hog plum, cucumber, snake gourd, aubergine, pumpkin, squash, yam, trumpet flower, bean, sandal, sloe, garlic, onion and suchlike. But she does not discuss her assets with others or tell them about the advice given by her husband.
(26–30)

Among women of her class she stands out for her skills and her appearance, her dignity, culinary ability and entertainment. She estimates the household's annual income and adjusts the expenditure accordingly. From leftover food she makes ghee, oil and jaggery. From cotton she spins and weaves thread. She stores unused slings for carrying loads, cords and strings for tying and fastening, and tree barks for making ropes. She supervises the pounding and cleaning of rice and makes use of the chaff, the broken grains and, after cooking, of the gruel and the charcoal. She keeps track of the servants' wages and meals, of agriculture, animal husbandry and the upkeep of carriages. She also looks after the household's rams, cocks, quails, parrots, mynahs, cuckoos, peacocks, monkeys and deer. The daily income and expenditure are kept under scrutiny. Worn and old clothes are collected, cleaned or dyed, and gifted to servants as tokens of appreciation for their work, or utilized elsewhere. The jars for wines and spirits are stored and used; their purchase and sale are supervised, together with the resultant expenditure and revenue.
(31–35)

Her husband's friends are honoured appropriately with gifts of flowers, perfume and betel leaf. She is deferential in attending to her parents-in-law, never contradicting them, speaking little but never curtly, and refraining from loud laughter. She further treats those whom they like or dislike in the same way. (36–37)

She is modest in her enjoyments, considerate to servants and does not give anything to anyone without informing her husband. She also monitors servants in their work and honours them on festival days. Such is the life of the only wife. (38–41)

During the Husband's Absence*

When he is travelling and away, the only jewellery she wears is that which signifies that she is married. Awaiting his news, she keeps fasts dedicated to the gods and looks after the household. She sleeps at the feet of the elders, does her work with their advice and endeavours to acquire and preserve things her husband would like. Her expenditure on daily needs and special tasks is appropriate and she does not forget to complete the works her husband had begun. Her visits to her own kinsmen are confined to occasions of joy and grief. Even then she goes with someone from her husband's household, without any change in her style of dressing during his absence, and does not stay out too long. (42–45)

Her fasts are undertaken with the elders' permission. All selling and buying is carried out through honest and dependable servants, so that the assets can be augmented and the expenditure minimized as much as possible. On her husband's return, she first lets him see her in the common garb she had worn while he was away. Then she prays to the gods and offers him some gifts. Such is her life during his absence. (46–47)

There are two verses here:

> Such is the life that she should lead
> as an only and devoted wife,
> though she may be a woman of
> good family or one remarried,
> or even a concubine.
> For women of such noble conduct
> gain Dharma, Artha, also Kama,
> a place of honour and a husband
> who will never take another co-wife.
> (48)

CHAPTER TWO:

One of Several

The Senior Wife*

The addition of a co-wife takes place when the first is frigid, promiscuous or a bringer of bad luck; if she cannot have children or repeatedly has only daughters; or if the husband is fickle-minded and capricious. The first wife should preclude this from the beginning by demonstrating her devotion, virtue and proficiency. If she cannot have children, she herself urges the husband to take a co-wife. (1–2)

The new co-wife would naturally try to create a situation of predominance for herself. So, the senior should treat her like a sister. She prepares her for the night with many efforts, and makes sure that the husband knows this. She ignores her hostility or any haughtiness springing from her good fortune.
(3–4)

She disregards any negligence shown by the new co-wife in relations with their husband. When she thinks that the new one will herself correct it, she advises her with care. She also briefs her confidentially, but within the husband's hearing, about the special techniques of love-making which please him.
(5–6)

She shows no discrimination against the new wife's children. Her servants she treats with the utmost sympathy. She displays affection for her friends, and for her relatives an extreme respect, even more than for her own kin.
(7)

If the senior has been followed by several co-wives, she cultivates the one immediately after her. She also encourages quarrels between the co-wife whom the husband likes most of all and the one who was previously in that position, sympathizing with the latter and uniting the others to denigrate the current favourite as a wicked person, without herself getting into the argument.
(8–11)

Further, she promotes friction between the favourite and the husband, taking her side and egging her on to make the quarrel grow or, if it is subsiding, to light a spark herself. But if she thinks that her husband still cares for her, she works on her own for peace between the two. Such is the conduct of the senior wife.
(12–15)

The Junior Wife*

The junior should regard the senior co-wife as a mother. Without informing her, she does not make use even of what she has received from her own kinsfolk. All her activities are carried out under the senior wife's supervision and it is with her approval that she sleeps with the husband. She does not tell others what the senior has told her and displays greater regard for the latter's children than for her own.
(16–21)

She attends more on the husband in private but does not tell him how she herself suffers because of the co-wife's hostility to her. Secretly she tries to get some special token of the husband's esteem, telling him that she indeed lives for such support. But, after getting it, she never reveals it to others out of pride or anger, for a woman who betrays the husband's confidence earns only his contempt.
(22–27)

The junior wife, says Gonardiya, should seek the husband's attention secretly for she should fear the senior wife. But if the senior is unlucky enough not to have any children, she should treat her with compassion, and also urge the husband to do the same, while supplanting her and assuming the role of an only wife. This concludes the conduct of the junior wife.
(28–30)

The Remarried Woman*

The remarried woman is a widow who, tormented by the weakness of the flesh, again attaches herself to some man endowed with good qualities and given to enjoyment. According to the followers of Babhravya, she may also be a woman who on her own leaves a husband, saying he is worthless, and desires another man.

(31–32)

In attaching herself to another man, she is in fact looking for happiness. And that is what marks her, says Gonardiya, for the totality of happiness lies in good qualities as well as their enjoyment. It depends on whatever is in keeping with one's own inclinations, according to Vatsyayana.

(33–35)

The remarried woman may want her relatives and husband to provide enough to meet her expenses for drinking parties, excursions, faith offerings and gifts to honour friends. Or she may do this from her own resources. The jewellery she wears is her husband's or her own, there being no rules for gifts made out of love. But she should return all other things given by the former husband if she leaves him of her own will. If she is turned out, she need give nothing back.

(36–39)

She treats the new husband's home as if she were its mistress. With his other wives of good family she is affectionate, with his servants considerate, and with his friends gay but always respectful. Adept in all the arts, she also knows more about them than her husband. If there is an occasion to quarrel, she reproaches him herself. But in private she follows him in the sixty-four arts of love-making. To her co-wives she does personal favours. To their children she gives ornaments, treating them like their superior and showing her approval with gifts of clothes and cosmetics. To his servants and friends she gives even more. And she is always ready for company, drinking

parties, picnics, excursions and other amusements. Such is the way of the remarried woman.
(40–44)

The Unlucky Wife*

The unlucky wife, neglected by her husband, is oppressed by her co-wives. Among them she should seek the support of one for whom their husband cares most. To her she demonstrates the pleasurable arts and skills she knows, for her misfortune leaves no room for keeping secrets.
(45)

She acts the nurse for the husband's children, cultivates his friends and makes her devotion to him known through them. She takes the lead in religious rites, vows and fasts, and is considerate to the servants without putting on too many airs.
(46–49)

In bed, she turns herself on in ways that suit the husband's inclinations. She does not reproach him or act contrary, and if any co-wife quarrels with him she helps in reconciling them. If there is some woman he secretly wants, she brings them together and keeps it confidential. In effect she so conducts herself as will make the husband think her chaste, undeceiving and devoted to him. This is the way for an unlucky wife.
(50–54)

Life in the Harem*

The preceding sections are also pointers to the life in a royal harem.
(55)

The women chamberlains or guards present garlands, pomades and garments to the king, informing him that they have been sent by the queens. The king takes them and gives in return garlands and flowers as signs of his acceptance of the offerings. In the afternoon he sees all the ladies of the harem in a single group. He is duly accoutred for the occasion, as are they. He talks and jokes with them, in keeping with their status and the time they have been in the harem. In the same way he meets his remarried women, and also the courtesans and the dancing girls who stay in the harem, each in their assigned quarters.
(56–62)

In the afternoon, when the king has risen after a siesta, the keeper of the roster informs him of the lady whose turn it is to be with him that night, the one who had the previous turn and any who are in their fertile period. The servants of each follow the keeper and present to the king containers of pomade stamped with the women's seal rings. The one picked up by him indicates whose turn it will be.
(63–64)

All the ladies of the harem are honoured appropriately with drinks during festivals, concerts and exhibitions. But they do not go out, nor do women from outside come in, except those of known purity, so that the activity inside remains undisturbed. This concludes the life in the harem.
(65–66)

The Man with Several Wives*

There are some verses on this:

> Having many wives collected,
> a man should treat them equally:
> not slighting any one of them,
> nor putting up with their deceptions.
> (67)

> The games one plays in making love,
> the special features of her body,
> her intimate talk and any reproach,
> he must not tell the other wives.
> Nor must he give an opening
> to one against another wife,
> or any cause or reason for it.
> And if one of them complains, she should
> be held to be the one at fault.
> (68–69)

> One by private confidences,
> another by public honour,
> and one by showing great respect:
> thus he pleases all his women.
> Each one he needs to gratify
> with garden outings and enjoyments,
> with gifts and honours to her kin,
> and the pleasures of love in privacy.
> (70–71)

The girl who will control her temper
and act in keeping with these precepts
will have the husband in her power
and be supreme among the co-wives.
(72)

BOOK FIVE

Wives of Others

CHAPTER ONE:

The Natures of Women and Men

Thoughts on Adultery

We have already discussed the reasons why men have sex with wives of others. Is it doable? Is it safe? Is it permissible? What of the future and one's livelihood? These aspects need to be considered from the very beginning.
(1–2)

It is to save his own self from being consumed by desire that a man makes advances on another's wife. He does this when desire is perceived to be rising from one stage to another. These stages are ten. Their signs are: pleasure at sight; obsession of the mind; beginnings of a longing; sleeplessness; loss of weight; revulsion from other subjects; loss of shame; hysteria; fainting and eventually death.
(3–5)

The Nature of Women

Many teachers have said that a young woman's character and truthfulness, her purity and attainability, and the intensity of her sexual impulse are indicated by her appearance and physical characteristics. But these can be misleading, according to Vatsyayana. It is only from her gestures and signals that a woman's nature can be gauged.
(6–7)

According to Gonikaputra, on seeing an attractive man a woman will desire him. So too will a man on seeing a woman, though he may go no further for some reason. But women are different. A woman just desires: she does not consider if it is right or wrong. She may not take the initiative for other reasons and, if propositioned by a man, it is in her nature to turn off even if she desires him. Therefore she needs to have repeated advances made in order to be won over.
(8–12)

The Nature of Men

As for a man, even if he desires a woman he may desist from proceeding further due to considerations of virtuous behaviour and nobility of conduct. With such thoughts he cannot be won over easily, despite the woman's advances. His own are made for no particular reason and, after making one, he may not repeat it as, once he has had her, he becomes indifferent. There is a common belief that a man looks down on a woman who was easily had, and wants one who is hard to get.
(13–16)

Why Women Get Turned Off*

Here are the reasons for a woman turning away from a man's advances. Love for her husband. Concern for her children. Onset of age. Desolation due to some grief or sorrow. Absence of opportunity. Anger: 'His proposition is an insult.' Indecision: 'He is unfathomable.' The belief that 'This has no future. He will go away as he is infatuated with someone else.' Alarm:

'His intentions are too blatant.' The thought that 'He cares more for his friends and will tell them all.' Suspicion: 'He is not serious.' Diffidence: 'He is too grand.' The doe woman's apprehension: 'He may be too strong and his sexual impulse too fierce.' Shyness: 'He is so urbane and expert in all the arts.' The thought that 'He always treated me like a comrade.' Revulsion: 'He has no thought of the proper time and place.' Lack of respect: 'He is disgraceful.' Contempt: 'He does not realize it even when I signal him.' The elephant woman's concern: 'He is a hare type and his sexual impulse may be dull.' Sympathy: 'He is out of his mind and may get into trouble.' Disgust at noticing her own bodily defects. Fear: 'I will be thrown out if my family gets to know.' Scorn: 'He is old, gone grey.' Doubt: 'He has been put up by my husband to test me.' And finally, her concern for virtuous conduct.

(17–42)

Overcoming Resistance*

From the very beginning a man should pre-empt whichever of the aforesaid elements he notices. Those relating to the nobility of her temperament, by exciting her passion. Those arising from her sense of inability, by pointing out solutions. Those due to her great respect for him, by greater intimacy. Those caused by her lack of respect, by his boldness and skill, and those because of his own disrespect, by humbling himself. Her fears he should relieve with assurances.

(43–49)

The following men are generally successful with women: one familiar with the *Kama Sutra*; an expert teller of stories; an associate since her childhood; one in the prime of youth; one who has gained her trust through games and other amusements; a doer of what he has been asked; a good talker; a doer of what she likes; a former messenger of another lover; a knower of her vulnerabilities; one sought after by the highest women; one secretly involved with her girl friend; one known to be lucky in love; one who grew up with her; a pleasure-loving next-door neighbour; a similar servant; the husband of her nurse's daughter; one recently engaged; a generous spender who likes picnics and pageants; one so hot and strong that he is called a bull; someone of daring and courage; one who surpasses her husband in learning and looks, in virtues and enjoyment; and a man who lives and dresses well. (50)

Easy Women*

Just as a man considers the attainability of a woman from his perspective, so should he from hers. The women who can be had without effort or merely by making an advance are such as these: she stands in the doorway; keeps looking out of her house at the highway; spends time chatting at a young man's home next door; is always staring; throws sidelong glances when noticed by a man. She has been superseded by a co-wife for no cause; hates her husband, who hates her too; is uninhibited; and has no children. She stays all the time with her relatives and her children have died. She is fond of parties and wants to be friendly. She is the wife of an actor; a young girl whose husband is dead; a poor woman who likes to enjoy herself; the wife of the eldest of several brothers; a vain woman with an inferior husband; a woman proud of her skills and distressed at her husband's stupidity, ordinariness and greed. Or, she may be

a woman approached by someone who had made efforts to get her when she was a girl, but somehow did not; or by someone whose mind and disposition, intellect, perception and background are similar to hers. Or a woman who is by nature partial to the man; has been dishonoured by her husband for no fault and denigrated by co-wives of comparable looks; and whose husband is always travelling. Or one whose husband is jealous, dirty, a pimp, impotent, a procrastinator, cowardly, a hunchback, a dwarf, deformed, a jeweller, rustic, sick, old or malodorous.
(51–54)

There are two verses on this:

> Desire springs from nature itself,
> but actions make it grow;
> it becomes imperishable when
> the mind is of anxiety freed.
> (55)

> On knowing well his own ability
> and a woman's tell-tale signals
> a man may cut through all the causes
> of her reserves and have her.
> (56)

CHAPTER TWO:

Gaining Access

Through a Messenger

Many teachers have said that a virgin girl can be won more easily through a man's own advances than through a woman messenger acting as the go-between. With other men's wives, they say, it is more delicate and those women are better won through the female messenger. There is also a common belief that women who are daring for the first time to venture into an affair and are uninhibited in talking about it can be seduced by a man on his own, while the opposite kind of women need going through a messenger. According to Vatsyayana, one's own efforts are more effective in all cases, depending of course on one's abilities. It is only when the latter are inadequate or there are difficulties that a woman messenger is required.
(1–3)

Getting Acquainted

A man wishing to make an advance needs first to get himself acquainted with the woman he desires. His meeting her can either be natural or it can be contrived. The natural way is in the vicinity of his own house. The contrived one can be at the house of a friend, a kinsman, a high official or a doctor; or on the occasion of a wedding or a sacrificial ceremony, a festival or some calamity, an excursion to a park or other such events.
(4–5)

When she sees him, he gazes at her steadily while making signals. He pats his hair down, snaps his fingers, tinkles his ornaments, bites his lower lip and makes other such signs. As she looks on, he talks about her with his companions on some pretext, displaying his liberality and sense of enjoyment. Reclining by a friend's side, he may stretch his limbs, yawn and raise an eyebrow, speaking slowly while listening to her talk. Using words with double meanings, he addresses a child or another person, indirectly expressing his own desire for her. And, in another signal, he kisses and embraces the child, gives it a betel leaf with his tongue and tickles its chin with his forefinger, doing all this at appropriate moments. Or he may fondle the child seated in her lap, give it a toy then pull it away and, being near her, start up a conversation. Becoming friends with someone well known to her, he uses that person to gain access and talks within her hearing about the *Kama Sutra*, of course without looking at her. As their acquaintance grows, he finds excuses for further interaction by lending her things like betel nuts and perfumes for long or short periods, taking the opportunity to ask for them later. He also arranges intimate get-togethers for her at a private place, even with his own wives.
(6–10)

To meet her regularly and gain her confidence, when she needs something from the goldsmith, the jeweller or the gem-cutter, the dyer with colours of indigo or safflower, he arranges the business himself through his own servants. Organizing such work provides occasions for long and public meetings with her so that one transaction will lead to another. Thus, he makes it known that the production and application, the knowledge and the means of acquisition of the works, materials and skills she may want are all within his capacity to deliver. He also discusses with her and her associates how people tested the

quality of work in the past, and arranges for her to act as the arbitrator in specific matters, saying 'It will be marvellous,' if she questions him. Such is getting acquainted.
(11–18)

Making a Pass*

Once he has got to know the woman and she has indicated her feelings through gestures and expressions, the man may advance with the methods used in the case of a virgin girl. There they are generally subtle, for virgins have not yet had sex, but with other women who have, the very same advances can be quite open. So, when her reactions are clear and her feelings revealed, they share and enjoy each other's possessions. These can be things like valuable perfumes, scarves, flowers and rings. On the way to a party, he takes a betel leaf from her hand, asks for a flower from her hair and gives her a precious perfume or some other desirable object with his nail or teeth marks on it as a token.
(19–22)

Dispelling her diffidence with more and more advances, he gradually goes with her to secluded places. They embrace and kiss. They exchange betel leaves and other things, in the course of which he touches her in her private parts. Thus are advances made. But, while making up to one woman one should never do so with another. And if there is one with whom a man has earlier had an affair, he should placate her with things she likes.
(23–26)

There are two verses here:

> One should never make a pass
> at a woman, even though

she is easy to be had,
when her husband is seen to be
going about with someone else.
Conscious of his own reputation,
a wise man will not think about
a woman suspicious by nature,
well protected or afraid,
or living with her mother-in-law.
(27–28)

CHAPTER THREE:

Appraisal of Feelings

Need to Appraise

One needs to study a woman's behaviour when making a pass at her. This also gives a measure of her feelings in responding to the advance. If she does not manifest any, a female messenger or go-between may be required to win her over. If she does not react, but meets the man again, it shows that she is in two minds. He can then hope to win her by slow degrees. (1–3)

While not responding overtly to his advances, if she still lets herself be seen all dressed up by the man, and comes to him so attired, it is an indication that she is available, but by force when they are alone. If she does not yield despite permitting many advances for long, she is a flirt. Then, as the human heart is always changeable, one must break off relations in order to have her eventually. Another woman avoids the man making advances. She neither comes to him nor turns away. This is because she is conscious of her own importance. Such a woman is not easy to get just by cultivation. She needs winning over through a messenger or go-between who knows her weaknesses. The woman who rebuffs an advance rudely deserves to be dropped, but she can still be won if, despite her rudeness, she is in search of pleasure. A woman in two minds will allow the man to touch her on some pretext, as if she did not notice it. Such a one can be had with patience and persistence. (4–10)

Further Indicators

Pretending to be asleep, a man puts his hand on the body of a woman lying by his side. Though liking it, she too reacts as if asleep, but pushes the hand away on seeming to wake up. This shows that she wants further advances. This can also be seen by his putting a foot on hers and, progressively, by embracing her while feigning sleep. She may then get up as if it was too much. But if she acts normally the next day, it shows that she still wants the advance to continue. On the other hand, if she will not allow him to see her, she needs to be won through a messenger. Then, even after not having seen him for a long time, she comes to meet him as before, and signals to him with gestures and expressions so that he may resume his approach. (11–15)

A woman may encourage a man even without being approached. She reveals her limbs when they are alone and speaks tremulously. Her breasts heave. Perspiration appears on her face, hands and toes. She offers to massage his head and thighs, and does so eagerly, massaging him with one hand while

embracing him with the other, and seeking to be touched herself. Acting wonder-struck or just tired, she then stays still, with both her arms touching his two thighs or her forehead resting on them. Asked to massage him in the groin, she does not object but just puts one hand there, without moving it. And when he squeezes it hard between his legs, she removes it only after much time. Having thus accepted the advance, she then comes again the following day to massage him once more.
(16–19)

Or, she may neither become too intimate with the man, nor avoid him. For no reason she displays her feelings openly when they are alone. Otherwise she hides them. She may then be having an affair with a personal attendant and wishing to continue it even after being approached. In that case she needs to be won through a go-between who knows where she is vulnerable. But if she still turns away, then she is a doubtful case. Such is the appraisal of feelings.
(20–23)

There are some verses on this:

> Get to know her, first of all,
> then start a conversation,
> and mixed with talking there can be
> exchange of hints and signals.
> From her responses, if he sees
> acceptance of his approaches,
> a man may then no more hesitate
> but go all out for the woman.
> A woman who already shows
> her feelings through her gestures,
> needs to have a swift response
> at the very first meeting.

And she who openly reacts,
even to a gentle hint,
longs for sex, it should be known,
and can be had in a moment.
Women are winnable, it is clear,
but here are subtle methods shown
to deal with ladies unexpressive,
not bold, yet with enquiring minds.
(24–28)

CHAPTER FOUR:

The Go-Between's Role

The Need

A woman one meets rarely, and who has with her gestures given encouraging signals which she never did before, needs to be approached through a female messenger acting as the go-between. (1)

The Role

The go-between wins the woman's confidence by being agreeable. She entertains her with smooth talk of beauty treatments and what others are doing, and with tales told by bards and stories of romantic affairs, while flattering her with praise for her good looks, knowledge, courtesy and character. 'How could someone like you have such a husband?' she says to

make her feel a tinge of regret, 'Good lady, he is not fit even to work as your servant!' And she speaks to her at length, with feigned sympathy, about his sexual dullness, jealousy, dishonesty, ingratitude, aversion to enjoyment, stinginess, whimsicality and other defects, harping in particular on those which she considers most hurt the wife. Thus, if the latter is a doe woman, the husband is not faulted for being a hare man; this is said only if she is a mare or an elephant woman.
(2–8)

According to Gonikaputra, the woman's feelings may be in a delicate state as she dares for the first time in her life to have an affair. After winning her trust, the go-between tells her of the suitor's accomplishments, his suitability and longing for her. And, as the woman reveals her true feelings, the messenger plots her own way to her goal. 'Listen, good lady,' she tells her, 'this is an extraordinary situation. That man is from a good family. Seeing you has turned him mad. He has a gentle nature and the poor fellow has never been smitten before by anyone else. Now he is even prepared to die for you.'
(9–12)

She repeats this story on the following day, noting the sparkle it has brought to the woman's eyes and face, to her voice and gaze. And as the latter listens, she tells her the well-known and now pertinent tales of Ahalya, Avimaraka, Shakuntala and others. She speaks about the man's virility, expertise in the sixty-four arts and his luckiness in love. She talks of his secret affairs with some celebrated women, which may or may not have taken place.
(13–15)

Then she observes her expression. The woman looks at her and speaks with a smile; invites her to take a seat; asks her where she has been, slept and eaten, what she has been doing;

and opens up to her when they are alone. She starts narrating stories, sighs thoughtfully and yawns, gives her a present in token of her love, invites her to select festivals and lets her go with the promise that they meet again. 'You speak so nicely,' she says at the end, 'then why do you tell me such terrible things?' And she talks of her suitor's duplicity and fickleness. Without herself mentioning how she earlier met and interacted with him, she looks to the go-between to refer to it and, when the latter speaks about the man's wishes, the woman laughs them off without any definite response. On getting such signals, the go-between should bolster them with further reminders about the man, his love for the woman and his various qualities. (16–31)

According to Auddalaki there is no role for a go-between when two people neither know nor have received signals from one another. The followers of Babhravya say that there is a role, even when they do not know each other, if one has signalled to the other. According to Gonikaputra, although they may not have exchanged signals, there is still a role if they know each other. In the view of Vatsyayana there can be a role even without any mutual acquaintance or exchanges. It depends on their confidence in the messenger or go-between. (32–35)

Sending Love Tokens

The go-between shows the woman gifts sent by the man to steal her heart: a betel leaf or a pomade, a necklace, a ring or a garment. The container of each carries signs made with the man's teeth or nails to convey his intent. The garment is marked with a supplication made in saffron. She also shows the woman

leaves cut in various shapes to indicate the man's feelings and, concealed in ear ornaments and chaplets, written messages expressing his wishes. The woman then sends gifts in return. Such mutual exchanges, carried out with trust in the messenger, lead to a meeting.
(36–41)

Meetings

According to the followers of Babhravya, meetings may take place on occasions such as visits to temples, expeditions, garden picnics, water sports, weddings, sacrificial ceremonies, festivals, spectacles and also at times of trouble like fires, robberies and armed invasions of the country. Gonikaputra says that homes of girl friends, nuns, women mendicants and ascetics are convenient places for a meeting. The woman's house itself is always convenient, according to Vatsyayana, if one knows how to get in and out, has thought out reactions to any trouble and if entrance and exit is secure even at unpredictable times.
(42–44)

Kinds of Go-Between

There are different kinds of women messenger or go-between: one fully mandated; one with only a limited mandate; just a carrier of letters; one acting for her own self; one acting for a fool; a wife who acts the messenger; one who stays mute; and one like the wind.
(45)
The fully mandated go-between is one who has understood the end desired by both the man and the woman, and then uses her

own head to bring it about. She is generally used by people who already know and have talked to each other, but may be used by a woman even when they have not, or by a couple similar and suited to each other, and mutually curious even though unacquainted. (46–49)

The go-between with a limited mandate knows of a part of the affair and the advances made, and works to bring about the rest. She is used by couples who have noted each other's signals but can meet only rarely. The letter-carrier merely brings messages. She is used just to fix a rendezvous by couples who already know and have deep feelings for each other. (50–53)

Then there is the go-between who pursues her own interest. She is sent by another woman but, as if unknowingly, herself propositions the man. She tells him she dreamt he was sleeping with her, complains that he called her by his wife's name and uses this as a pretext to show that she feels jealous. She also gives him something with her nail or teeth marks on it, saying, 'I had decided from the beginning to present this to you.' And, when they are alone, she quizzes him, 'Who is more enjoyable, I or your wife?' Such a woman is to be seen and received privately. On the excuse of having brought a message from another woman, she uses the opportunity to harm her and herself seduce the man. It is said that men also do this when acting the messenger for another man. (54–57)

There is another type of woman, one who worms her way quietly into the confidence of a man's naive wife and asks her about his activities. She offers instruction in love-making, in dressing to send signals and in feigning anger, telling her, 'This is what you should do.' She makes nail and teeth marks on the wife's body, sending in this way her own signals to the man.

Such is the messenger acting for a fool. A man may give his responses similarly. Or he may get his own naive and foolish wife to gain the other woman's confidence so as to send her signals and make his abilities known to her. Here the wife acts as a messenger, and signals can also be received through her. (58–60)

Then a man may send a young servant girl, who knows no wickedness, as an innocent medium, with a garland or an ear ornament containing a secret note or a nail and teeth mark. This is the mute messenger, and he can also ask for a reply to be sent through her. Finally there is the messenger like the wind, wholly detached from the message she carries. Containing previously arranged meanings and marks which others cannot divine, it may also have both a common and a double intent. The reply, too, can be requested through her. These are the different kinds of women messengers. (61–62)

There are some verses on this:

> A widow, a female fortune-teller,
> a servant maid, a beggar woman,
> and a woman artisan
> are quick in winning confidence
> to act the role of go-between.
> (63)

To put it briefly,

> She gets the husband to be hated,
> extols the other person's charms,
> reveals, even before other women,
> his marvellous ways in sex.

She speaks of the man's affection,
his skill in making love,
his being sought by better women
and still remaining true.
With her clever use of words
a messenger can turn around
even an unintended meaning
in words uttered by mistake.
(64–66)

CHAPTER FIVE:

Sex and Men in Power

A Warning

Kings and their ministers
do not enter others' homes
as many people watch the way
they behave and do the same,
just as all the world gets up
when the rising sun it sees
and, on beholding it go down,
also turns to rest.
(1–2)

They should therefore not do anything which is improper, both because it is not done and because it would invite censure. But if it becomes inevitable, they need to resort to expedients.
(3–4)

Available Women

Young village headmen, officers and sons of farm superintend-
ents can have village women with just a nod. Their hangers-on
call such women wanton. They can be had when engaged in
unpaid labour, in filling granaries, bringing in and taking things
out, cleaning house, working in the field, collecting cotton, wool,
flax and tree bark, getting thread, and in the sale, purchase or
exchange of goods. Thus are dairy maids used by the keeper of
cows; widows, orphan girls and homeless women by the spin-
ning-master; women who roam the streets by the police chief
who knows their secrets because of his own wanderings at night;
and those who buy and sell by the man in charge of the market.
(5–10)

Women in cities, suburbs and market towns generally go to
the home of a man in power on occasions like the eighth and
the full moon night and the spring festival for social gatherings
with the ladies of his harem. After the drinking party there,
these city women separately visit the chambers of the harem
ladies they know, where they are welcomed and offered drinks,
sit and talk before going home in the evening.
(11–12)

A royal servant maid, who already knows the woman
desired by the man in power, is sent to talk to her on such occasions and to prepare her with a display of beautiful things. She
would have spoken to the woman even earlier at her own
home. 'I will show you some beautiful things at the royal palace at such and such a gathering,' she would have said while
fixing a time. 'I will show you the floor outside, inlaid with
coral, the altar made of gems, the orchard, the bower of grape
vines, the secret passage in the palace walls, the lake pavilion,

the pictures, domesticated animals, mechanical toys, caged birds, tigers and lions, and other things I earlier mentioned.' And, when they are alone, she tells her of the lord's passion for her, describes his skill in making love and gets the woman to agree without telling anyone else about the proposal.
(13–19)

If the woman does not agree, the lord then comes himself and propitiates her with courtesies and civilities. Having had his way, he lovingly sends her off. If her husband is fit to be favoured, he has that man's wives always come to the harem at suitable times, when the royal servant maid is sent as before.
(20–21)

Alternatively, the woman wanted by the lord is cultivated by another lady from the harem who sends her own servant to her as their friendship grows. And when they meet, the woman is honoured, offered drinks and the royal servant maid despatched as before. Or, if the woman he wants is well known for skills like music, the lady from the harem formally invites her to give a performance, and when she comes the royal servant maid is sent as before.
(22–23)

If the woman desired is the wife of someone in a state of fear because of an imminent problem, a beggar woman tells her: 'There is such and such a lady in the harem who has influence on the king. She listens to me and does what I ask of her. As she is kindly by nature, I will find some way to go to her myself and arrange your entry there. She will take care of your husband's great problem.' Convincing her thus, she takes her in twice or thrice, and the lady in the harem gives her assurances which please her no end. Then the royal servant maid is sent as before.
(24)

The same approach can be made with wives of men who are in search of a job, harassed by ministers, forcibly arrested, with few legal resources, dissatisfied with their standards of living, seeking royal favour, wishing for a place in official circles, troubled by their kinsmen or wanting to trouble them, seeking to pass information, and others wanting something.

(25)

Or, if the woman desired by the lord is involved with someone else, he can just have her taken into custody, appointed as an attendant and gradually introduced into the harem. Or her husband is accused by a spy of being against the king and she is arrested as the spouse and brought into the harem in this way. Such are the secret methods. They are generally used by princes.

(26–27)

But a man in power should never enter another person's home. It is said that the Kotta king, Abhira, did so and was killed by a washerman engaged by the owner's brother. Jayasena, the king of Kashi, was killed by the chief of his cavalry.

(28–29)

Desires can also be pursued openly, in keeping with local practices. Among the people of Andhra, a newly married local girl goes with some presents on the tenth day to the royal harem and returns only after having been enjoyed. Among the people of Vatsagulma, the wives of ministers and other lords go at night to service the king. Among those of Vidarbha, the ladies of the harem keep beautiful local girls with them for a month or half a month on the pretext of their affection for them. In the land of Aparanta, people gift their good-looking wives to ministers and kings, just as tokens of their love. And, in that of Saurashtra, women of the city and the countryside enter the

royal household individually, and in groups, for the king's pleasure.
(30–35)
There are two verses on this:

> These, and many other ways
> of having wives of other men,
> are prevalent in different places,
> propagated by men in power.
> But a king who is devoted
> to the people's welfare, will not
> ever use these methods and,
> quelling the enemies six within,
> conquer all the earth.
> (36–37)

CHAPTER SIX:

Women in the Harem

Their Sex Life

For the women of the harem, there is no meeting men because they are guarded, and no satisfaction because there is only one husband in common for many wives. So, they simply use other means to give pleasure to one another. Dressing up the daughter of a nurse, a girl friend or a servant girl as a man, and equipping her with something of appropriate shape, a tuber, root, fruit or a dildo, they then relieve their own desires. They also lie on statues of men where the penis is not clearly visible.

Kings who pity them will go with a dildo to many such women in one night, even without feeling any passion, although if it is the appointed turn of a woman they love or one who is in her fertile period, they then give vent to their own desire. These are eastern practices. As with women, men deprived of sex too are known to relieve their desires with objects other than a vagina, with animals, images of women and by straightforward masturbation.

(1–5)

The women of the harem often have their servant girls bring in gentlemen disguised in female garb. The daughters of their nurses, too, if they are well introduced inside the harem, try to get these men in by pointing out possibilities for the future. They tell them how easy it is to enter and of the points of exit, the vastness of the building, the carelessness of the guards and the frequent absence of the servants. But they should not make the mistake of getting people in under false pretences.

(6–9)

Advice to Outsiders

According to Vatsyayana, even if the harem is easily accessible, a gentleman should refrain from entering it because of the great likelihood that this could be disastrous for him. However, he may enter if he has been invited by the women many times, has understood the method of getting out which they have suggested and has assessed what he will gain from the visit. He needs first to investigate all aspects thoroughly: the harem's exit, its surrounding pleasure park, the openings in its high walls, whether the guards are indeed few and careless, and the

king is away. Depending on the possibilities, he could then come out every day.
(10–12)

On some pretext he makes the acquaintance of the guards outside and gets to recognize the king's spies. He makes out that he is attached to a servant maid inside who is aware of his desire. Grief-stricken at not meeting her, he asks the other women who go in to act as his messengers. In case the agreed messenger woman cannot go in, he stands where the woman he wants can see and signal to him. Here too he gives the excuse of the servant maid to the guards. And when his gaze meets that of the woman he desires, he signals to her with gestures, draws suitable pictures at the spot where she is looking, writes bits of songs with double meanings there and places near it toys and balls he has marked, together with a ring.
(13–19)

Methods of Entry

Only after noting her response does he try to enter. He finds out the passageways she uses and hides himself there in advance, or enters at a time fixed by her, dressed as a guard. Or, he enters and comes out covered in a bedsheet or a cloak. Or, he makes himself invisible with the magic trick of 'fold-unfold'. This is how it is done. Take the heart of a mongoose, the eyes of a snake, the fruit of fenugreek and a long gourd plant. Cook them on smokeless fire. Then grind equal parts into a paste. When this is applied to the eyes, both one's form and one's shadow disappear. Or, he comes in at the moonlight festival with the lamp-carriers through an underground passage.
(20–26)

This is how it happens:

> When objects are being removed
> and drinks are being brought inside
> for a feast of revelry
> and servant girls are in a rush;
> when the house is being shifted
> and there is a change of guard;
> when expeditions to parks occur
> or when they are coming back;
> and when the king himself proceeds
> on a journey that is long:
> it is then that, generally,
> a young man enters and exits.
> And, some women of the harem,
> knowing each the other's wish,
> in what should be done, united,
> get the rest to join them too
> through corrupting one the other,
> so that the man, resolute in his
> dedication to a single goal,
> can then never get betrayed
> but may straightaway enjoy
> the fruit that he desires.
> (27–28)

Regional Practices

In Aparanta the denizens of the harem are not too well guarded, and the women visiting the royal palace themselves bring good-looking men inside. The Abhira women fulfil their desires with

the harem guards themselves, who are known as the warriors. The women of Vatsagulma get sons of gentlemen inside dressed as errand girls, along with those girls.
(29–30)

In Vidarbha, the sons of denizens visit the harem whenever they wish and sleep with all women except their own mothers. In the kingdom of women the ladies of the harem do this only with their visiting kinsmen and relatives and not with others. In Gauda the women of the harem do it with brahmins, friends, attendants, servants and slaves; and those in Sindhu with porters, artisans and others of this ilk who are not barred from the harem. In the Himalayas bold men bribe the guards and enter the harem in a group. In Vanga, Anga and Kalinga the brahmins of the city, charged with making gifts of flowers, go into the harem with the king's knowledge. There they talk with the women who are behind a curtain, and a union takes place in due course. In eastern lands nine or ten women get together and keep a young man hidden among them. Thus are the wives of others seduced and such is the life of the women in a harem.
(31–38)

Guarding the Harem*

One's own wives need to be guarded for these very reasons. Many teachers have said that guards for the harem should be appointed only from people of proven loyalty in matters of sex. But they could let someone in out of fear or greed. Therefore, according to Gonikaputra, they should also be of proven loyalty in aspects apart from sex. According to Vatsyayana, though loyalty is a sacred duty, even so people abandon it out

of fear. They should as such be tested also for their adherence to virtue.
(39–42)

According to the followers of Babhravya, one's own wives should also be tested to ascertain their purity or impurity. This can be done through women who keep their own intent secret and will report on what others say. But just because such wicked people succeed with young women, according to Vatsyayana, one should not let the innocent be tainted for no reason. What ruins women is: too much partying; absence of discipline; the husband's wilfulness; unrestrained behaviour with other men; staying away from home; living abroad; loss of livelihood; association with loose women; and the husband's jealousy.
(43–45)

A man who knows this book of rules,
and has seen the methods used
to target other people's wives,
will not get cheated by his own.
But do not go for others' wives:
these methods are but optional,
with clearly visible dangers,
and they go against the pursuit
both of virtue and of wealth.
This disquisition has been made
for the welfare of all men
and for keeping all wives safe.
It should not be understood
as meant for spoiling people.
(46–48)

BOOK SIX

The Courtesan

CHAPTER ONE

Helpers, Worthwhile and Avoidable Clients, Motivations

General

Sleeping with a man is basically a source of pleasure and a means of livelihood for courtesans. Done for pleasure, it is natural. Doing it for gain is artificial even though a courtesan makes it appear natural as men feel confident with women who are moved by desire. To this end she displays an absence of greed and, to safeguard her future, refrains from going for easy money.
(1–6)

Helpers

A courtesan is just like something on sale. She is always well presented as she looks out at the high street, visible but not too exposed. She finds friends who can help to attract the man she wants and keep him away from other women, people through whom problems can be solved, purposes accomplished and who will not be treated with contempt by her clients. These people are city guards, officers of law courts, astrologers, bold men, soldiers, men with knowledge similar to her own, men adept in the arts, professional companions, hangers-on and jesters, garland-makers, perfumers, wine-sellers, laundrymen, barbers, beggars and others suited for particular jobs. (7–9)

Worthwhile Clients

The clients entertained merely for money are these: some-one free of encumbrances; a young man recently come of age; a rich man; one with a visible source of income; one holding a position of authority; one with easy money; one given to com-petition; a man with a steady income; one proud of his luck in love; a braggart; a eunuch wanting to be taken for a man; a man wanting to do better than his equals; one of a liberal dis-position; one with access to the king or his minister; a fatalist wanting to spend his money fast; one who does not care for money; one who disobeys his elders; a man held as an icon by his kin; the only son of a rich man; a religious student; a man with secret desires; a soldier; and a physician. (10)

But courtesans also looking for pleasure and celebrity go for clients of quality. And these are: a man of noble birth; a learned man; one who knows the proprieties; a poet or a skilled story-teller, eloquent and eminent; an adept in the various crafts; a man respectful of elders; an ambitious and resolute man; one steadfast in loyalty; one free of envy, generous and caring for his friends; one fond of large and small get-togethers, of shows, drinking parties and literary games; a man free of disease and bodily defects, full of life and not addicted to drinking; a friendly man, as strong as a bull in sex; one attractive to women, who flirts with them but is not in their control; a man

of independent means; one who is never coarse, jealous or apprehensive.
(11–12)

As for the qualities in a courtesan, she has beauty, youth, sweetness and auspicious body marks. She likes men for their merits, not merely their money, and enjoys sex with love. She has a steady mind, does not dissemble, appreciates refinement and is never disagreeable. She also delights in parties and the arts. In addition, she possesses the following general qualities. Intelligence, character and proper behaviour. Straightforwardness, foresight and gratitude. An avoidance of controversy, an understanding of the right time and place, and courtliness. She refrains from looking miserable, from excessive laughter, malicious talk and slander, from anger, avarice, insensibility and capriciousness. She speaks when spoken to. And she is adept in the *Kama Sutra* and its ancillary skills.
(13–14)

Clients to Avoid

The inverse of the aforementioned good qualities are defects. The clients to be avoided are as follows. Someone with the wasting sickness, with worms in his stool and breath which smells of crows. Someone in love with his spouse. One who is coarse in speech, mean, pitiless, disowned by his elders, and a thief. A man duplicitous, addicted to black magic. One who is uncaring of honour or dishonour, who can be bought even by his enemies and who is completely shameless.
(15–16)

Motivations

According to many teachers, the reasons why women sleep with men are: love, fear or gain; competition and settling scores; curiosity and partiality; exhaustion or a sense of duty; fame, compassion, the word of a friend, resemblance to someone dear; embarrassment, gratification or relief of passion; kinship, living in the same house, constant togetherness and concern for the future. According to Vatsyayana the reasons are gain, avoidance of loss and pleasure. Gain, being the principal reason, should not be constrained by pleasure. As for fear and the other reasons, one should examine how weighty or not they may be. This concludes the consideration of Helpers, Worthwhile and Avoidable Clients and Motivations for having them. (17–20)

Getting a Client*

Even when approached by a worthwhile client, a courtesan does not accept him straightaway, for men hold in contempt what is easy to get. She sends her principal servants, or masseurs, singers and jesters devoted to him, to find out his feelings and, in their absence, she sends professional companions and such people. Through them she can learn about the man's purity and impurity, if he is passionate or not, attached or indifferent, generous or miserly. Once the prospect is clear, she arranges a tryst through a professional hanger-on or pander. (21–24)

The companion brings the man to her house, or her to his, on the pretext of watching a fight between quails, cocks or

rams, of hearing a parrot and a mynah bird talk, or attending some other spectacle or exhibition. On his arrival she offers him a love-gift, something which will please him and arouse his curiosity, saying 'This is specially for you to enjoy.' She extends courtesies and entertains him with amusing conversation. And, after he leaves, she immediately despatches a servant maid who will talk to him with a smile and carry a present for him. Or she goes herself with a companion under some pretext. Such is the winning of a client.
(25–30)

Here are some verses on this:

> To the visiting man she offers,
> lovingly, a betel leaf,
> a flower garland, some refined
> pomade, and talks about the arts.
> She gives him some personal things
> and exchanges them with his;
> by herself, thus making known
> her readiness to sleep with him.
> And, once they become intimate,
> with love-gifts, suggestions and
> actions having just one meaning,
> she gives full pleasure to that man.
> (31–33)

CHAPTER TWO:

Pleasing the Lover

Advice in Brief

Once she takes up with a lover, the courtesan acts like an only wife in order to please him. To put it briefly, she gives him pleasure but is not attached to him, even though she behaves as if she is. (1–2)

Role of the House Mother

The courtesan represents herself as dependent on a mother who is hard-hearted by nature and thinks only of money, or, in her absence, on an adopted mother. Neither cares much for the lover and tends to force the daughter to come away from him. At this the courtesan exhibits displeasure and dejection, fear and embarrassment, but she never disobeys her mother's orders. If she has some reason for not going to the lover, she feigns a sudden, singular illness, nothing repulsive, just invisible and temporary, and makes that a pretext, sending him leftover flowers and betel leaves through a servant girl. (3–11)

Pleasing the Lover

While making love, she marvels at his techniques, acts like his pupil in the sixty-four arts and repeatedly practises his lessons.

Her behaviour accords with his personality when they are alone. She tells him her desires, but conceals any abnormalities in her secret places. In bed, she never ignores his turning towards her and reciprocates his touching her private parts.
(12–19)

She kisses and embraces him when he is asleep, and watches him when his mind is preoccupied. When he is on the road, she gazes at him from the house but, if he notices her, looks bashful to preclude any impression of cunning. She hates what he hates, likes what he likes, takes pleasure in whatever pleases him and follows him in grief and joy. She is curious about his women but never angry for long, though she suspects others for the nail and tooth marks on his body, even when she herself has made them. Her own passion she never expresses in words, but makes it known through gestures and signals or, wordlessly, by the pretence of being drunk, unwell or dreaming.
(20–26)

When her lover talks about his own admirable deeds, she grasps the point of his words and takes it into account while praising him. But she replies only if he has shown himself to be devoted to her. She concurs with all that he says except for the subject of his other wives. When he sighs or yawns, stumbles or falls, she wishes him good health. If he sneezes, cries out or seems astonished, she exclaims 'Live long!' When he is out of sorts, she pretends to be unwell too.
(27–32)

She does not praise others in front of her lover, nor disparage them for faults similar to his. What he gives, she wears, but does not dress up or eat if he blames her for no reason or is in some trouble. She then grieves with him and prefers to pay for a royal exit permit and leave the country with him, for her life is meaningful only because she has him. When he comes into money, achieves a desired goal or recovers from some illness, she makes an offering earlier vowed to her favourite god.

(33–40)

She eats little and is always well turned out. In her singing she includes her lover's name and lineage. When she is tired she draws comfort from his hand, putting it on her breast or brow as she falls asleep. She also sleeps sitting in his lap, and follows him when he leaves her.

(41–43)

She wants to have a child by him and does not wish for a life longer than his. When they are alone she does not talk of things unknown to him. She dissuades him from making vows and keeping fasts, saying 'Let this be on me!' and, if she cannot, does the same herself. If he disagrees, she tells him that even he cannot stop her.

(44–47)

She makes no distinction between what is his or hers, does not go to parties and other gatherings without him and boasts of wearing his used flower garlands and eating his leftover food. She praises his family, his character, artistic skills and learning, clan and class, wealth and land, friends and merits, age and sweetness of temper. If he knows singing and such arts, she urges him to indulge in them.

(48–52)

She goes to him without concern for danger, cold, heat or rain, saying, 'May he alone be mine, even in the next life.' She conforms to his favoured tastes, feelings and attitudes, and is suspicious of magic and sorcery. Always arguing with her mother on the subject of going to him, if she is forced to go to someone else she asks instead for some poison, a dagger, a rope, or will just not eat, to kill herself. This she conveys to her lover through confidential servants or directly so that he may understand her conduct, for she never argues with her mother about money matters or does anything without consulting her. (53–61)

When her lover goes away on a journey, she makes him swear that he will return quickly. During his absence she abstains from makeup, or wearing jewellery except for good luck, such as a single conch-shell bangle. Remembering their time together, she visits fortune-tellers and soothsayers and expresses envy of the heavenly constellations, the sun, the moon and the stars, for he can see them but not her. 'May we be united!' she says on seeing him in a dream, but when alarmed by some bad omen she performs the rites of propitiation. On his return, she prays to Kama, the god of love, makes offerings to all the gods, has a filled jar fetched by her girl friends for thanksgiving and puts out the ritual food for the crows. But all these, except for the crow ceremony, are done only after they have first made love. (62–71)

To a devoted lover, she talks of following him in death. The signs of such a lover are that he trusts her feelings, has the same attitudes, does her bidding, is free of suspicion and does not care for wealth. All that has been said here is meant to cite examples from the rules of Dattaka. What is unsaid, one should practise in accordance with local customs and the nature of men. Here are two verses on this:

> As they are subtle, excessively greedy,
> and their nature is little known,
> women's feelings are hard to fathom,
> even by those whom they desire.

They want someone, then turn indifferent,
give delight, and then abandon,
they even extract all one's money:
women just cannot be understood.
(72–76)

CHAPTER THREE:

Making Money

Expedients

Getting money from an infatuated man can be both natural and contrived. According to many teachers, a courtesan need not contrive expedients if she can get as much as she wants or more by being natural. According to Vatsyayana, a man will give even the double of the amount agreed if he is induced with expedients.
(1–3)

And these are the expedients for getting his money. To repay loans taken for the procurement of ornaments, cooked and uncooked food, drinks, flowers, clothes, perfumes and other material, or for the refund of a monetary deposit. By praising his wealth to his face. On the pretext of goodwill gifts needed for festivals connected with vows, tree plantations, orchards, temples, lakes and parks.
(4–6)

She says that her jewellery was stolen by the guards or by robbers when she was on her way to him. Or, that a fire in the house, the breach of a wall, or some carelessness has caused a

loss of property and of the jewellery borrowed for or belonging to the lovers. She also informs him through her confidential servants of the expenses she has incurred in going to him. She takes a loan for him, and has an argument with her mother about the resultant expense. She declines to go to friends' parties as she has nothing to give them as a present when, as she had already mentioned, they had brought valuable gifts for her. Then she suddenly stops her daily routine.
(7–13)

She gets artisans to make things for the lover, does favours to ministers and physicians for having some work done and helps the lover's friends and benefactors in their difficulties. There are also the pretexts of work needed in the house, a ceremony for the son of her girl friend, a pregnancy, an illness and helping another friend in trouble. She talks of having to sell part of her jewellery for the lover's sake, showing to a merchant what she wears, together with the household utensils and furniture. And on occasions when similar household effects of other courtesans are pooled together, she takes the best of them for her lover's house.
(14–20)

She never forgets to praise in public the favours she received earlier from her lover, but gets her confidential servants to talk within his hearing of the larger rewards earned by other elite courtesans. Then she tells them, in his presence and with some embarrassment, of her own much greater rewards irrespective of whether she ever got them or not. While she openly refuses previous clients who try to re-establish a liaison with a larger offer, she also tells her lover of the generosity of his rivals. And, when she thinks that he will not come back, she goes begging to him like a child. These are the expedients for getting money.
(21–26)

Signs of the Lover Cooling Off*

A man's loss of interest can always be deduced from the changes in his attitude and the look on his face. He gives her less than usual or an extra amount. He makes contact with her rivals. Pretending to do one thing, he does something else. He cuts off his normal routine, forgets a promise or says he never made it and speaks with his people in a sign language. He sleeps somewhere else on the pretext of some work for a friend and talks privately to the servants of his former mistress.
(27–35)

Before he can become aware of it, the courtesan should then take possession of all his money, under whatever pretext, and get a creditor to seize it forcibly from her. If this is disputed, it can then be taken to court. This concludes the lover's cooling-off.
(36–38)

Getting Rid of Him*

A lover who did favours in the past, and is still attached, needs to be looked after even though he now yields but little fruit. But one without resources and any means should be got rid of by some expedient, or with the help of another man. And these could be the ways. Doing something he dislikes. Practising what he condemns. Curling her lip in a sneer. Stamping her foot on the ground. Talking of things he knows nothing about. Expressing not wonder but contempt at what he does not know. Deflating his pride. Associating with his superiors. Ignoring him. Criticizing those with faults like his. And staying away from him.
(39–41)

She gets agitated by his behaviour when making love. Does not offer him her mouth. Shields her pelvic zone. Is disgusted at the wounds he makes by scratching and biting. Crosses her arms to prevent his embrace. Stiffens her limbs and crosses her thighs. Wants to sleep. And, when she sees that he is tired, she urges him on, mocks him when he cannot do it and turns off when he wants to. Noticing his arousal even during the day, she goes out to be with a crowd.
(42)

She misconstrues what he says. Laughs when he has not said anything funny and, when he has, chuckles and speaks about something else. With a side glance at him, she looks at and slaps a servant. She interrupts what he is saying with another story, talks publicly about his lies and the vices he cannot give up and exposes his secrets through a servant girl. She does not see him when he comes, and she asks him for the impossible. The release then comes by itself. This is what Dattaka has said about the client.
(43–44)

There are two verses on this:

> After having checked him out,
> to get together with the client,
> pleasing him when he is hooked
> and relieving him of his wealth,
> finally, to let him go:
> this is the courtesan's way.
> With the methods here prescribed,
> the courtesan in her liaisons
> is not excessively cheated
> by the clients, and collects
> a large amount of money.
> (45–46)

CHAPTER FOUR:
Reunion with an ex-Lover

His Background

When a courtesan discards an existing lover after squeezing him dry, she may renew a previous liaison. Her former lover too may have lost money, but in case he is still wealthy and loves her, he is worth getting back.
(1–2)

However, it needs to be considered how he strayed elsewhere. Depending on the circumstances, there could be six possibilities: (i) he left her on his own initiative, and has left the other woman too on his own; (ii) he left both on being turned out; (iii) he left her place on his own, but the other on being turned out; (iv) leaving her on his own, he has taken up with another woman; (v) he was turned out from her place, but the other he left on his own; (vi) turned out from her place, he has taken up with another woman on the rebound.
(3–9)

Is He Worthwhile?

If he is negotiating a return after leaving both places of his own accord, it shows that he does not care for either, is fickle-minded and not worth getting back. But leaving both after being sent away indicates a certain constancy of mind. If the other woman offended him even when he had the wherewithal and threw him out because she wanted much more from him, and if the

courtesan feels 'He will give me a lot because he is angry,' he is worth trying to get back. If he was rejected because of his poverty or miserliness, he is not a good prospect. On the other hand, if he left the courtesan on his own and the other woman on being asked to leave, he should be accepted provided he gives an additional amount of money as an advance.
(10–13)

'He left from here on his own, is at another place and now negotiating a return.' Such a case deserves consideration. 'He comes because he wants something special. He wishes to come to me because he did not find it there. He wants to know me better and will pay because he still loves me.' Or, 'having seen the other woman's flaws, he will now notice my superior qualities and give me much more.' Or, 'his mind is like a child's, unfocussed.' Or, 'he has too many affairs.' Or, 'his passion is as fleeting as the colour of turmeric.' Thinking of all this, she may or may not have him back.
(14–16)

'He left from here on being turned out. He is leaving the other woman of his own accord and now seeking a return.' This also needs consideration. 'It is because he loves me that he wants to come back. He will give much because he thinks of my good qualities and takes no pleasure in that other woman.' Or, 'I threw him out unjustly in the past. He harbours a grudge and now cultivates me in order to take it out on me.' Or, 'he wants to win my confidence, so that he may use it to get back the money I had been able to extract from him.' Or, 'he intends to abandon me after making me break with my present lover.' A man with such a disagreeable mindset is not worth taking back. He could, however, become worthwhile with a change of mind in the course of time.
(17–20)

Rationale for Reunion

The foregoing applies to a man the courtesan had turned out, who is now with another woman and seeking a return. She may herself negotiate with him from among those who send feelers to her. 'The reason for which I discarded him was false,' she considers. 'Hence he strayed elsewhere. Now I need to make an effort to get him back. If he is talked to from this side, he will break off from the other and stop his payments there.' Or, 'he is making good money now, his house is bigger. He has won several appointments. Separated from his wives, divided from his parents and brothers, he is free of encumbrances.' Or, 'by making up with him, I will be able to get a rich lover to whom he is connected.' Or, 'his wife insulted me and I will instigate a quarrel between him and her.' Or, 'his friend is in love with my co-wife who hates me. Through him I will cause them to split.' Or, 'I will get him into trouble by exposing his frivolity and fickle-mindedness.'
(21–30)

Methods

So, she gets her counsellors and other aides to tell him that he was turned out because of her mother's wickedness, and that she was helpless even though she loved him; that she feels no desire for her present lover, sleeping with him but also hating him. Her aides remind him of her love with some memento, a souvenir of some favour he did to her. This concludes the reunion with an ex-lover.
(31–34)

Summation

According to many teachers, as between someone who has never been her lover, and one who has, the latter is better for the courtesan. His disposition is known, his passion tested and he is easier to serve. According to Vatsyayana, it is almost meaningless to consider a former lover as one who will provide some money: all of it has already been squeezed out of him. It is also hard to get back his trust. A new lover, on the other hand, can be easily pleased. Even so, there are exceptions which depend on the nature of the man. (35–37)

There are some verses on this:

> This is why the courtesan seeks
> reunion with a former lover:
> to split him from another woman,
> or the woman from the man,
> or to hurt her present beau.
> (38)

> A man attached excessively
> gives much money out of fear:
> he fears she'll go to someone else,
> so her deceits will disregard.
> She greets the man still unattached,
> ignoring one in love with her,
> and when a messenger comes
> from another well-known man,
> she makes a rendezvous with him
> who had made the first approach,
> not breaking off the old connection

or discarding former lovers.
The man attached and in her power
she consults, and carries on
with another man from whom
she gets money, then returns
to give pleasure to the first.
(39–42)

A clever woman, initially,
will consider future prospects and
the gains, the pleasure maximum
and the friendship she can get
in reuniting with a previous lover.
(43)

CHAPTER FIVE:

Particular Profits

Kinds of Profit

The courtesan need not limit herself merely to one client if she
can profit from many every day. She considers the place, the
time and the situation, her own qualities and charms and how
they compare with those of other courtesans. Then does she
establish a price for the night, send messengers to the client or
herself call those who may be connected with him. To gain a
very large profit she may go, even two, three or four times, with
just one client and act like his wife.
(1–4)

According to many teachers, when there are several clients who offer the same profit, the one who can deliver the thing she wants is obviously preferable. And he, according to Vatsyayana, is the one who pays in gold. For everything can be done with gold and it cannot be taken back. Gold, silver, copper, bronze, iron utensils, furniture, bedsheets, cloaks, special clothes, aromatic substances, pungent spices, pots, ghee, oil, grain and different cattle: each of these is preferable to the one which follows it. When the people and the things they offer are similar, a choice can be made on the basis of a friend's advice, one's immediate needs, future prospects, the client's qualities and of course love.

(5–8)

Passionate, Generous and Grateful Lovers

As between a passionate and a generous lover, the generous one is obviously preferable, according to the teachers. It is, of course, possible to inspire generosity in a passionate man. According to Vatsyayana a passionate lover can be generous even if he is a lecher, but a generous one cannot merely be pressed into passion.
(9–11)

The teachers further say that a rich lover is preferable to a poor one because, as between someone just generous and a person who will serve your purpose, the latter is obviously better. However, one who serves a purpose thinks he has done what he had to after doing it just once, whereas the generous lover does not dwell upon what he gave in the past. This is the view of Vatsyayana, though here too preference depends on immediate needs.

(12–14)

Many teachers say that, as between a grateful and a generous lover, the latter is clearly to be preferred. In Vatsyayana's opinion a generous lover, even though he may have been cultivated for a long time, will not consider the courtesan's past services if he hears of even a single deception on her part or if she is falsely maligned by rival courtesans. This is because generous givers are usually haughty, plain-spoken and somewhat disdainful of others. The grateful, on the other hand, care about past services and will not break off suddenly. Moreover they will not be poisoned by falsehoods as they are familiar with the courtesan's character. Here, of course, preference depends upon future needs.
(15–19)

Other Considerations

The teachers say that, as between the counsel of a friend and the acquisition of wealth, the latter is obviously preferable. According to Vatsyayana money can be gained in the future too. As for the friend, if his advice is disregarded he may be turned off from helping again. Here also it is preferable to meet an immediate need. The courtesan can mollify the friend by showing him some work which must be done while saying 'your advice will be carried out tomorrow,' and take the money available straightaway.
(20–23)

As between making a profit and avoiding losses, the first is patently preferable according to many teachers. But Vatsyayana says that the extent of profit has a limit; as for losses, once they commence none can know where they will end. Preference

depends on their relative importance, but preventing a loss is preferable to a doubtful gain.
(24–27)

The Long Term

From the excess over their profits, the elite courtesans spend money on building temples, pools and gardens; constructing fire altars on drained land; donating thousands of cows to brahmins through the intermediary of trusted people; arranging prayer offerings for the gods or providing money to bear that expense. Courtesans of the middle variety, those who subsist on their beauty, spend their excess on jewellery for adorning their limbs; enlargement of their home; and the improvement of its decor with valuable utensils and servants. And the lowest, the pot-carrier servant women, spend it on wearing fresh, clean clothes every day; eating and drinking to their fill; always using fragrances and the betel leaf; and on sporting jewellery partly made of gold. This is the way that all courtesans, even those of the middle and lower kinds, use the excess of their profits, in the opinion of many teachers. According to Vatsyayana, however, the profit from this livelihood is never constant, as it depends on the place and the time, prosperity and power, love and local predilections.
(28–32)

With a well-intentioned man, the courtesan may settle even for a very small profit. She may also do so if she wants to keep a client away from someone else; or steal another's lover; or deprive another courtesan of some gain. She may think that she will improve her own position, desirability and future prospects by going with that particular client; or want to get his help in pre-empting a loss; or wish to hurt a former lover; or have in view a previous favour; or simply be in search of pleasure. But she will take nothing at all if she is looking to her future, and turning to that client in the hope of averting some loss. (33–34)

However, she will seek an instant gain if she thinks: 'I will leave him and take up with another person'; or 'he will leave me'; or 'he will go back to his wives'; or 'he will liquidate some loss of his'; or 'his supervisor, master or father will come and restrain him'; or 'he is capricious.' On the other hand, if she concludes: 'he will get the reward promised by the king'; 'he will obtain a post or position'; 'this is the time for his pay'; 'his ship is coming in'; 'his holding or harvest is ripe'; 'what he did will not be lost', or 'he is always true to his word' – then, considering her own future prospects, she will act like a wife. (35–36)

There are some verses on this:

> It may be her future needs,
> or those which are for here and now,
> but she avoids, keeps far away
> from those cruel royal favourites
> whose money comes through wicked means.
> There are some, refusing whom
> is disastrous, while going with
> them could lead to greater heights:
> approach them under some pretext,
> grab them, even with some effort.
> And those who proffer countless wealth
> when pleased, even a little bit,
> broad-minded men of great energy:

they should be gone after, pursued
even at her own expense.
(37–39)

CHAPTER SIX:

Gains and Losses, Consequences and Doubts

Causes of Losses

Working for gain can also lead to losses, with other consequences and doubts. Losses accrue from a weakness of the
mind; from an excess of passion or conceit, duplicity or upright-
ness, trust or anger; from carelessness and recklessness; and
because they are fated to happen. They result in fruitless work
and expense. Future prospects are ruined. The inflow of money
gets reversed. That which was gained is dissipated. The mind
becomes obtuse and withdrawn. The body becomes prone to
injury and accident: falling down, losing hair, getting hurt.
Therefore losses should be avoided from the very beginning,
ignoring even some substantial gain.
(1–4)

Definitions

There are three kinds of gain: of wealth, of virtue and of pleasure. Losses, too, are three: of wealth, of virtue and of pleasure
which is repugnance. When the pursuit of one leads also to
another, that is a consequence. Uncertainty about getting a

result: 'will it happen or not' is a pure doubt, and 'will it be this or that' is a mixed doubt. The appearance of a second objective while pursuing the first is a double combination; and the appearance of several is a multiple combination. We will give examples of all these. The form of the three gains has already been discussed. That of the three losses is exactly the opposite. (5–12)

Examples

The courtesan obviously gains wealth in going with a man of the best class. She also has future benefits. Her desirability increases and she is sought by others. This is one gain which has the consequence of another. Consorting with someone merely for the money, however, is a gain without a consequence. (13–14)

Accepting from a lover money which belongs to someone else cuts into future possibilities as the money may get taken back; and if he is base and generally despised, going with him ruins one's future. This is a gain with the consequence of a loss. (15)

Going at one's own expense with some avaricious warrior, minister or other influential person who will not spend his money is not gainful. Even so, it may serve the purpose of solving a problem, removing the cause of a greater loss or creating an opportunity in the future. This is a loss with the consequence of a gain. (16)

The cultivation of a miser, who thinks himself good-looking, has no gratitude or is exceedingly duplicitous, will be fruitless. This is a loss without a further consequence. However, if he is

a royal favourite, cruel and influential, then not only is his cultivation fruitless but getting rid of him can also cause harm. This is a loss with the consequence of a further loss. The consequences of gaining virtue and pleasure can be determined in the same way, and each can be combined with the other. So much for consequences.
(17–20)

Kinds of Doubt

'Even if he is satisfied, will he pay or will he not?' This is a doubt about the gain of wealth. 'His wealth wrung out, he gives nothing. Unable to get more, if I throw him out, will it be right or will it not?' This is a doubt about the gain of virtue. 'If I go with an attractive servant or some other lowly person I find, will it conduce to pleasure?' This is a doubt about getting pleasure.
(21–23)

'Will an influential but base person who remains ungratified cause me a loss or not?' This is a doubt concerning loss of wealth. 'If a lover who gives absolutely nothing is discarded and then dies, will I have done wrong or not?' This doubt concerns the loss of virtue. 'Will my passion turn into aversion if I am unable to get the person I want even after I have expressed my feelings to him?' This is a doubt concerning repugnance or the loss of pleasure. This concludes simple doubts.
(24–26)

Now, the mixed doubts. 'Will gratifying a visitor whose character is unknown but who is influential or recommended by a lover, lead to my gaining or losing money?' This is one form of doubt. 'The passion of a learned priest or a religious celibate, an ordinand or one under holy vows, or a wearer of

sacred marks, has been aroused on seeing me. So much so that he is ready to die. Will it be right or will it be wrong to go to him out of kindness as advised by a friend?' This is another. 'People are undecided if a particular man has good qualities or not. Will going with him without consideration of this aspect give pleasure or will it cause aversion?' This is yet another kind of doubt. All these can be further combined with one another. This concludes mixed doubts.
(27–31)

Combinations

Now the double combinations. When money is gained from an affair with someone, and simultaneously from an existing lover because of his rivalry with that man, that is a double gain. When one's own money is spent on an affair with no returns, and an offended existing lover takes back what he paid, that is a double loss.
(32–33)

When there is uncertainty whether an affair will result in any gain or not, and also whether the existing lover will give anything in rivalry, this is a twofold doubt about gaining wealth. When she has an affair at her own expense with the thought, 'will my former lover harm me out of anger or not?' or 'will that offended lover take back the money he had given to me?' this is a twofold doubt concerning a loss. Such are the double combinations according to Auddalaki.
(34–35)

According to the followers of Babhravya: 'She gains from going to the man and also gains from a lover to whom she does not go.' This is a twofold gain. 'There is a fruitless expense in going to the man and an irreconcilable loss in not going.' This is a twofold loss. 'Going to the man will cost nothing, but it is uncertain if he will pay or not. Also, will the existing lover pay or not pay without my going to him?' This is a twofold doubt concerning a gain. 'Going to the man involves expense. Whether the former lover, influential and frustrated, can then be got back is uncertain. So too it is if he will harm me out of anger at my not going to him.' This is a twofold doubt concerning a loss.

(36–40)

A combination of the foregoing shows six kinds of mixed doubt: gain on the one side and loss on the other; gain on the one side and doubtful gain on the other; gain on the one side and doubt about loss on the other. Considering them with her helpers, the courtesan follows a course which provides for gain or its maximum possibility, or for the avoidance of some heavy loss. The gains and losses of virtue and pleasure can be inter-related, combined with each other and exemplified in this way also.

(41–43)

When several libertines get together to take one courtesan, that is a group possession. She consorts with them here and there, getting money from each one through their mutual rivalry. 'My daughter', she gets her mother to tell them, 'will go tonight with one who arranges such and such things for me for the spring and other festivals.' And she aims for what she needs, as going with her creates competition between these men.

(44–47)

Gain from one, gain from all; loss from one, loss from all; gain from half of them, gain from all; loss from half and loss from all. These are the group combinations. Doubts concerning gains and losses may be combined and computed as explained

earlier. So, too, can it be done for virtue and pleasure. This concludes the consideration of gains, losses, consequences and doubts.
(48–49)

Kinds of Courtesan*

Courtesans are of the following kinds: the pot-carrier servant woman; the attendant girl; the wanton; the promiscuous woman; the dancer; the woman artisan; the abandoned wife; the woman who lives on her beauty; and the elite courtesan. All of them need to give thought to compatible clients, helpers and to pleasing them; to methods of obtaining money, discarding clients and getting them back; to the consequences of particular profits; and to the consequences and doubts concerning gain and loss. This concludes the book on courtesans.
(50–51)
    There are two verses on this:

> Now men want pleasure
> and women want it too:
> here are precepts for women
> as wanting is mainly
> what these rules are about.
> There are women who care for passion,
> some others care also for wealth.
> Passion was discussed earlier,
> this book gives rules for courtesans.
> (52–53)

BOOK SEVEN

Esoteric Matters

CHAPTER ONE:

Looking Good and Other Subjects

The *Kama Sutra* has now been explained. But if one is unable to achieve the desired end by the methods suggested in it, the confidential prescriptions which follow may be used. (1–2)

Making Oneself Attractive

What makes one attractive are appearance, quality, age and liberality. A paste of rosebay, wild ginger and plum leaves can make one seductive. So can a salve for the eyes made by grinding these same herbs, putting the powder on a wick and burning it with myrobalan oil in a human skull. Also, a body lotion made by boiling hogweed, fleabane, silk cotton and red amaranth flowers with the leaves of the blue lotus in oil, or a garland strung with these flowers and leaves. (3–7)

Licking a paste of honey and ghee mixed with a powder of dried red and blue lotus and rose chestnut makes a person attractive. The same ingredients can be combined with rosebay, plum and bay leaf to make an ointment for application on the body. The eye of a peacock or a hyena, put inside a locket of gold and worn on the right hand, also renders one attractive. So too does an ornament made with a jujube berry or a conch

shell and used in the same way. Other similar methods from the *Atharva Veda* may also be followed.
(8–11)

Here is a method for increasing the desirability and good fortune of the master of a servant girl. When she has attained puberty, with his knowledge of methods and systems he keeps her away from other men for just one year. The charm of a girl thus secluded will make many people want ardently to have her, leading to their mutual rivalry. The master then bestows her on the man who gives the most among them.
(12)

The Courtesan and Marriage

An elite courtesan, too, guards her own daughter who has attained the prime of youth. She then invites young men similar to her child in skills, disposition and beauty, and tells them that whoever gives such and such specific things can have her daughter's hand. The girl also, acting as if her mother does not know it, encourages the interest of these rich sons of gentlemen. She arranges to meet them here and there, while taking art lessons, in music schools and at the homes of mendicant women. And the mother then gives her hand to the man who can provide whatever has been asked for. If she is unable to get as much as she expected, she may even supplement it with a part of her own money, declaring that it was given by that man for her daughter's hand or that she gave him her virginity. Alternatively, the courtesan gets them united secretly, as if without her knowledge, and then informs the courts that she has just learnt of it.
(13–19)

Elite courtesans also let the daughter go if she is of adequate age and beauty, her virginity has been lost to a girl friend or a servant and she has fully grasped the *Kama Sutra* and is well grounded in its methods through practice. These are eastern customs. For one year she stays faithful to the man who has taken her hand, and after that does what she pleases. But, if invited by him even after the year is over, she comes to him for the night though she may forsake some profit thereby. This is the practice a courtesan follows in marriage to enhance her attractiveness and good fortune. The same is the case with a girl who makes her living on the stage; but she is given to one who can promote her artistic career. This concludes the section on making oneself attractive.

(20–24)

Bewitching a Woman*

Sex with a woman when the penis is smeared with honey mixed with a powder of thorn apple, black pepper and long pepper will bewitch her into one's power. Using a powder made of wind-blown leaves, flowers left on a corpse and peacock bones has the same effect. So does a bath after putting on a powder of the remains of a kite which has died of natural causes, mixed with honey and gooseberries.

(25–27)

Cut bulbs of milkwort into pieces, dip them in a mixture of crushed red arsenic and sulphur, dry seven times, then powder them. Smeared on the penis with honey when having sex, this also bewitches the woman into one's power. Burnt at night, this powder makes the moon appear golden if it is looked at through the smoke. The same powder, when mixed with monkey shit and sprinkled over a virgin girl, ensures that she is not given to another man.

(28–30)

Coat bulbs of orris root with mango oil and place them for six months inside the hollowed-out trunk of a *sissu* hardwood tree. Taken out after that period and used as an ointment, this preparation, which is called 'dear to the gods', is said to bewitch women into one's power also. Another ointment, called 'dear to the demi-gods', is made by similarly placing thin pieces of catechu wood inside a hollowed-out tree for six months, where they acquire the fragrance of its flowers. Its use is said to have the same effect. A mixture of saffron and rosebay dressed with mango oil and kept for six months inside the hollowed-out trunk of an acacia tree makes an ointment called 'dear to the serpent-gods', which is said to have the same effect.

(31–33)

The bone of a camel, soaked in marigold juice and burnt, makes a collyrium which can be kept in a pipe. Applied with a pencil also of camel bone, this is said to be good for the eyes and to bewitch women into one's power. Collyrium for the eyes can be made in the same way from the bones of hawks, vultures and peacocks.

(34–35)

Enhancing Virility*

A man becomes as strong as a bull by drinking milk mixed with garlic, pepper and licorice and sweetened with sugar. Drinking milk boiled with the testicles of a ram and a goat and mixed with sugar is also a recipe for bull-like strength. Drinking it with milky yam root, dates and horse-eye beans has the same effect. So does milk drunk with seeds of long pepper and roots of sugar cane and milky yam.

(36–39)

Teachers have said that after eating to one's fill a porridge made of water chestnuts, lotus root and wild figs ground with dates and jujube and cooked with milk, sugar and ghee over a slow fire, one can make love with women endlessly. They say that a pudding made with the milk of a cow with a mature calf and lentil husk washed in milk and softened in hot ghee, when eaten with honey and clarified butter, also has the same effect. They further say that a man, having eaten to his fill cakes made of milky yam root, horse-eye beans, sugar, honey and clarified butter, can also make love with countless women.

(40–42)

The same result is obtained with rice grains soaked in the liquid of a sparrow's egg, cooked with milk and sprinkled with honey and clarified butter. Also, by eating to one's fill a pudding of unskinned sesame seeds soaked in sparrow's egg liquid, the fruit of water chestnut, lotus root and horse-eye bean, and powdered wheat and lentil, cooked with milk, sugar and clarified butter.

(43–44)

Teachers have said that two small measures each of clarified butter, honey, sugar and licorice, and larger measures of mead and milk, form a nectar of six elements, strong and tasty, which enhances virility and lengthens life. They also say that a concoction of molasses with asparagus and the dog-tooth plant, and a paste of long pepper and honey, when cooked in cow's milk and goat's ghee, makes a strong and tasty dish which enhances virility and lengthens life if taken every day in early winter. Further, that asparagus, dog-tooth and crushed lotus fruit, boiled in four times as much water to their natural consistency, make a strong and tasty dish which enhances virility and lengthens life when taken

on early winter mornings. The same result, they say, is obtained by taking two measures of equal parts combined of dog-tooth and barley powder on waking up every morning.
(45–48)

Methods which conduce to pleasure
may be understood and learnt
from the *Ayurveda* and
the *Veda*, other books of knowledge,
and from people one can trust.
But doubtful methods, do not use:
those which may the body harm
and those which involve killing creatures,
or the use of impure things.
Methods followed by good people,
which the brahmins recommend,
and all those who wish one well:
use, but with austerity.
(49–51)

CHAPTER TWO:

Revival of Passion

Manual Methods

A man unable to satisfy a woman with intense sexual impulses needs to use some method. At the start of making love, caress the opening between her legs with the hand. Enter when it has become wet and she is excited. This will revive her passion.

Oral sex revives passion in a man with dull sexual impluses, one who is old, fat or fatigued with love-making.
(1–3)

Artificial Means

Or use artificial devices. These, according to the followers of Babhravya, are made of gold, silver, copper, iron, ivory and buffalo horn. Those of tin and lead are soft, have cooling properties and provide better friction. According to Vatsyayana they can also be of wood, if that is preferred.
(4–7)

The inner side of the device should have the circumference of the penis. Its outer surface should be dimpled to make it rough. Two of these ring devices joined together are called a couple, and three or more, up to the length of the penis, are known as a crest. A beaded string wrapped around the penis according to its dimensions is a single crest. Another contrivance is called the armour or the little net. It is of the same dimensions as the penis, has openings at both ends and is fastened to the hips, with substantial hard cups for the testicles. In the absence of these, a squash, a lotus stalk or a bamboo section, well soaked in a decoction of oil and fastened to the hips, can also be used; or a string of smooth wooden pellets or gooseberry kernels. All these are discardable devices.
(8–13)

Perforation

It is said that a man cannot have real sexual union unless the penis has been pierced. Among the people of the south, the penis is pierced in childhood, just like the ears. A young man has it cut with an instrument and stands in water as long as the bleeding continues. To keep the opening clean he has continual sexual intercourse that very night. Then it is cleansed every other day with a decoction and enlarged by the insertion of reed and quince-wood pins of gradually increasing size. Cleansed with a mixture of licorice and honey, it is further enlarged with pins of lead and smeared with the oil of the marking nut. This is the method of perforating the penis. A variety of devices of different kinds can be placed in the opening thus made. These are the 'round', the 'round on one side', the 'little mortar', the 'little flower', the 'thorny', the 'heron's bone', the 'little elephant trunk', the 'eight rings', the 'bumblebee', the 'water chestnut' and others in keeping with the method and the act. This concludes our sixty-second subject, the revival of passion.

(14–24)

Enlarging the Penis*

Place the bristles of certain insects which are born from trees on the penis and message it with oil. Done for ten nights and then repeated, this will make the penis swell. Then lie face downwards on a string cot and let the penis hang down through it. This process should be concluded gradually, relieving any pain with cold salves. The swelling lasts for life. Libertines call it 'bristle-born'.

(25–27)

Massage with the juices of ground cherry, jungle yam, watermelon, aubergine, castor and heliotrope and with buffalo butter, one at a time, gives the penis an enlargement which lasts a month. Massage with a concoction of these cooked in oil

gives it for six months. So does massage or moistening with aubergine juice and oil cooked on a slow fire together with pomegranate and snake gourd seeds and red camphor. These and other methods may be learnt from trustworthy people. This concludes the subject of enlargement.
(28–31)

Various Prescriptions*

Sprinkle a mixture of powdered milkweed thorns, hogweed, monkey's shit and root of glory lily on a woman. She will not want sex with anyone else. In the same way, a man's passion disappears if he sleeps with a woman whose vagina has been smeared with a powder of rue, globe amaranth, marigold, iron, yellow amaranth and laburnum in a concoction of thickened rose apple juice. It also vanishes if he sleeps with a woman who has bathed in buffalo buttermilk mixed with bovine bile and a powder of mint and yellow amaranth.
(32–34)

A pomade or a garland made of the flowers of wild jasmine, hog plum and rose apple causes bad luck in the pursuit of love. An ointment of the root called the koel's eye will contract an elephant woman's vagina for one night. That of a doe woman will be widened by applying a powder of pink and blue lotus, wild jasmine and fragrant sal mixed with honey. Gooseberries soaked in a solution of milkweed, camphor and globe amaranth make the hair white. Bathing it in a mixture of henna, wild quince, frangipani, butterfly grass and the root of the smoothleaf tree turns it black again. The same combination, well cooked in oil, makes it turn black gradually. Lips reddened with lac turn white when moistened seven times with the sweat from the testicles of a white horse, but henna and the others already mentioned will restore their colour.

(35–42)

Coat a bamboo flute with a paste of mint, wild ginger, rose-bay, plum, deodar and prickly pear. When it is played, any woman who hears the sound will fall under the player's power. Eating or drinking anything mixed with the fruit of the thorn apple makes one go mad, but that person can be revived with old jaggery. Smear the hand with the shit of a peacock which has fed on yellow and red arsenic. Whatever is then touched will not be visible to others.

(43–46)

Water mixed with the ash of charcoal and grass turns the colour of milk. Iron pots become coppery when rubbed with a paste of yellow myrobalan, hog plum and the balloon vine. A lamp lit in balloon vine oil with a wick of cloth and sloughed snake skin will make long pieces of wood at its side look like serpents. And drinking the milk of a white cow which has a white calf gives fame and lengthens life, as do the blessings of respected brahmins.

(47–51)

Epilogue

This *Kama Sutra* is presented
in a form condensed with care
after studying earlier works
and noting their applications.
(52)

One who understands its essence
will look to virtue, wealth and pleasure,
his own faith, the world around him,
and not act just out of passion.
(53)

The various ways to enhance passion,
here put forward, as required,
at the same time, with due effort,
have here itself been proscribed too.
(54)

A practice should not be considered
just as 'prescribed by these precepts'.

For precepts have a general purpose
and practice follows specific cases.
(55)

Having learnt and pondered over
the precepts of Babhravya's school
in keeping with due procedure,
Vatsyayana made this *Kama Sutra*.
(56)

He composed it while observing
a celibate's life, in full meditation:
these rules are for life in this world,
they are not for passion meant.
(57)

One who understands the essence
of these precepts and safeguards
the state of Dharma, Artha, Kama,
in himself and in the world,
will his senses truly conquer.
(58)

Learned and adept in these,
looking to virtue, also wealth
and not seeking only pleasure
with a passion excessive,
he will succeed in what he does.
(59)

Notes

Notes to the Introduction

1. James McConnachie, *The Book of Love* (Metropolitan Books, New York, 2008)
2. ibid.
3. Sudhir Kakar, interview in *India Revisited*, ed. Ramin Jahanbegloo (Oxford University Press, New Delhi, 2008)
4. *Pancatantra of Visnuśarman*, ed. M.R. Kale (Bombay, 1912; reprint Motilal Banarsidass, Delhi 1982). This translation by A.N.D. Haksar.
5. ibid.
6. Kshemendra, *Chaturvargasamgraha* (2.24 and 3.3), in *Kshemendralaghukāvyasamgraha*, ed. V. V. Raghavacharya and D.G. Padhye (Osmania University, Hyderabad, 1961). This translation by A.N.D. Haksar.
7. Yashodhara in *Jayamangalā*, mentioned separately in this Introduction
8. A. K. Warder, *Indian Kavya Literature*, vol. 1 (Motilal Banarsidass, Delhi, 1974) and W. Doniger and S. Kakar, *Kamasutra* (Oxford University Press, New York, 2002)
9. Radhavallabha Tripathi, *Kamasutra of Vatsyayana* (Pratibha Prakashan, Delhi, 2005)
10. Patrick Olivelle, *Manu's Code of Law* (Oxford University Press, New York, 2005). In the present translation the word *shastra*

has been rendered as work, treatise, rules and science, depending on the context.

11. W. Doniger and S. Kakar, *Kamasutra* (Oxford University Press, New York, 2002)

12. A.K. Warder, 'Classical Literature', in *A Cultural History of India*, ed. A.L. Basham (Oxford University Press, Delhi, 1983)

13. For example, in Arjunavarma's thirteenth-century commentary on *Amarushatakam* (1 and 3), Mallinatha's fourteenth-century commentary on *Raghuvamsha* (19.16 and 19.31) and Kumbha's fifteenth-century commentary *Rasikapriya* on *Gitagovinda*. Also, *Kuttanimatam* (77 and 123) of Damodaragupta.

14. cf. 11 above

15. cf. 1 and 11 above

16. cf. 11 above

Notes on the Text

The figures at left indicate the page number of this work and, in the next column, the book, chapter and *sutra* number from the text of the *Kama Sutra* presented in this translation. The latter numbers are also given within individual notes to facilitate reference. The *sutras* have generally been shown in groups for ease of reading.

V refers to Vatsyayana, and K to *Kama Sutra*. M indicates *Manava Dharma Shastra*, also known as *Manusmriti* after the name of that authority. J refers to the commentary *Jayamangala* on K by Yashodhara. The numbers with it are of the *sutras* under comment. A stands for *Artha Shastra*.

3	1.1.4–5	The three ends of human life are explained further in Book One, Chapter Two of K, considered in Book Six, Chapter Six, and recalled in the concluding verses 53, 58 and 59 of the Epilogue in Book Seven, Chapter Two. Also discussed in the Introduction.

3	1.1.6–7	Manu, the son of the God of Creation, is the legendary author of M. This text exists though it may have undergone changes over time. It is now dated to *c*. 200 BCE–200 CE. Brihaspati was the guru of the gods. His abridgement of A is described in Book XII of the epic *Mahabharata*, but its text is no more available. A well-known work with the same name is extant and ascribed to the Mauryan minister Kautilya or Chanakya, *c*. fourth century BCE.
3–4	1.1.8–12	The great god is Shiva. His divine attendant Nandi is usually depicted as a bull in the god's shrines. The other writers mentioned here seem to be historical figures as most of them are separately mentioned in other texts, earlier or later than K. Their details are given in the Note on V's Predecessors.
4	1.1.13–14	The name V is omitted at this place in some recensions of K's text. But all name him as the author at 7.2.56. The text does not have the name Mallanaga which is mentioned in J (1.1.1 and 1.2.19) as the author's given name, V being his family name.
5	1.1.21	Though named as such here and in 6.3.30 the subject Getting Him Back is not described in the text, and hence excluded from our List of Contents.
6	1.1.23	The subjects earlier detailed in 1.1.15–22 actually total sixty-seven. They are not identified separately in the body of K's text, but J reconciles the number with V's total of sixty-four by omitting any separate identification of subjects at 1.5.1, 4.2.67 and

6.6.50. The aggregate of precepts or *sutras* seems to have been given as a round number here; the actual figure from the text comes to 1,683.

6-10	1.2.1–40	This outlines the overarching thesis within which K is expounded and which is reiterated at its conclusion in 7.2.53, 58–59: that Kama is but one of the three ends of human life and endeavour, and all need due consideration, as in 6.6.5–43. Also discussed in the Introduction.
9	1.2.26–29	Bali was the king of the demons and Indra of the gods. The former's elevation and downfall are a part of ancient mythology.
9	1.2.32–36	These examples of obsessive infatuation ending in disaster are taken from well-known stories in the epics *Ramayana* and *Mahabharata*.
12–13	1.3.13–16	The sixty-four arts refer both to social, domestic and artistic skills and to the techniques of love-making. The former are listed in 1.3.15 where the total could also be sixty-five. The latter, though never detailed in the same way, are mentioned in 1.3.22, 2.10.34–39 and 3.3.21.
13–14	1.3.17–18	The Sanskrit words for a courtesan are *veshya* and *ganika*. They are often interchangeable, but K uses the latter for women of a better class who also provided social and cultural company like the Japanese geisha or the Greek hetaera.
15	1.4.4	The betel leaf is still regarded as a stimulant, digestive and accompaniment to pleasur-

able pursuits. Touched with lime paste, catechu and other flavours and wrapped around finely chopped areca and other nuts, it is now normally consumed at the end of a meal.

16	1.4.8	His aides are further described at 1.4.31–35. The parasite has also been translated as a hanger on.
17	1.4.15	Sarasvati is the goddess of the arts and learning.
20	1.4.37	This could also be translated as refined (*samskrita*) and colloquial (*desha*) language.
21	1.5.3	The previously married woman is discussed further in 4.2.31–44.
29	2.1.1	J gives the numbers six, nine and twelve to suggest the dimensions, though it gives no unit of measurement for them. Some translators have equated them with four, six and nine inches.
30–31	2.1.13–18	See the Note on V's Predecessors.
33	2.1.33	J has calculated the total number of combinations as 729.
37–38	2.2.15–17	Also depicted in the famous temple sculptures at Khajuraho in Madhya Pradesh, India.
38	2.2.18–20	The two names suggest a mix which cannot be separated.
40	2.3.4–6	For Lata see Note on Place Names.
44	2.4.7–8	Explaining the reference to the left hand, J suggests that as the right is used much more its nails may get broken.

45	2.4.9–11	See Note on Place Names for Gauda and Maharashtra.
49–50	2.5.21–33	See Note on Place Names.
52–3	2.6.5–22	For Babhravya see 1.1.11–12 and Note on V's Predecessors. Indrani is the consort of Indra, the king of the gods. *Rigveda* 10.86 contains a dialogue on sexual intercourse in which she tells him how a man unable to satisfy a woman carnally can never be prosperous.
53	2.6.23	See 1.1.11–12 and Note on V's Predecessors for Suvarnanabha.
54	2.6.35	J quotes Gautama and Bhargava, two earlier authorities on Dharma, that sex in water is sinful.
55	2.6.45	See Note on Place Names for Bahlika and the kingdom of women.
58	2.7.24	J describes these in more detail. The 'wedge' is formed with the thumb overlapping the fore and middle finger of a closed fist. The 'scissors' involves the fingers spread out or curled and may be formed with one or both hands. The 'stabber' has the fist closed and the thumb protruding between the fore- and middle fingers. The 'pincer' seems similar, with the thumb between the middle and ring fingers.
58	2.7.25–30	Little is known about these incidents, which J also describes without shedding light on their location or time. A mythical chronology places Shatakarni of Kuntala as an Andhra king in *c.* seventh century BCE.

61	2.8.16	For Suvarnanabha see Note on V's Predecessors.
62	2.8.29–31	The box is described at 2.6.18.
64	2.9.1–5	According to J the third nature refers to eunuchs. The feminine ones have breasts and the masculine ones whiskers, among other characteristics. V uses the feminine gender in describing both. The word here translated as 'oral sex' is literally 'the one above'.
66	2.9.27–32	See Note on Place Names.
66–67	2.9.33–34	This verse occurs with slight verbal changes in the scriptural *smriti* text *Baudhayana Dharmasutra* (1.5.9). Its purport is also in M (5.130). Both predate K. Their argument is that the human or animal mouth, contact with which would otherwise be polluting, does not have this effect on given practical occasions.
68	2.9.43–45	In effect V describes the practice without giving a final opinion about its propriety.
69	2.10.5	For example at 2.2.14–17.
70–71	2.10.10–13	See Note on Place Names for Lata.
72	2.10.22	The Sanskrit word here translated as 'water-carrier' is also used at 6.6.50 to describe the lowest grade of courtesan.
73–4	2.10.34–39	See also the note to 1.3.13–16.
77	3.1.1	See Book One, Chapter Two for Dharma and Artha.
77	3.1.3	For Ghotakamukha see Note on V's Predecessors.

78–9   3.1.8–13   The verse about names is similar to the prohibition in M (3.9). The last sentence of this passage would seem to reflect V's own view.

79   3.1.15–19   The four rites mentioned in the penultimate sentence here are detailed in legal texts as also in M (3.27–30). They constitute the 'respectable' forms of marriage in which the bride is given away with due public ceremony by her parents or guardians to a groom of choice. There are four other recognized forms: *Asura* (by sale), *Gandharva* (a love match), *Rakshasa* (by capture) and *Paishacha* (by deception). All are mentioned at 3.5.12–30, but not named except for *Gandharva*, which is recommended.

79–80   3.1.20   Verse-capping or improvising a line to complete a stanza is one of the sixty-four arts mentioned in 1.3.15.

87   3.3.21   See 2.10.34–39 for the sixty-four techniques.

89   3.3.32   Later works on erotics also give ages for these female categories. For example, the *c.* sixteenth-century *Anangaranga* (4.1) classifies a girl as between eleven and sixteen years, a young woman as from sixteen to thirty years and a mature woman as from thirty to fifty-five years.

89–90   3.4.1–9   The 'touch' and other embraces are described at 2.2.6–13.

91   3.4.36   A woman taking the initiative to get married is in keeping with the injunction in M (9.90–91).

92   3.4.40–41   See 3.3.25–30.

95	3.5.1–2	The love story of Shakuntala is recounted in the epic *Mahabharata* and is the subject of a famous play by Kalidasa. It is an example of the *Gandharva* marriage mentioned below.
95–7	3.5.12–24	See note to 3.1.15–19. This portion describes the *Gandharva* form of marriage with variants. It is essentially a form based on the mutual attraction of the two parties and without any role for their families.
97	3.5.25–27	See note to 3.1.15–19. This portion describes the *Paishacha*, which is considered as the worst form of marriage in legal texts. The last sentence describes the *Rakshasa* form.
97–8	3.5.28–30	This makes clear V's preference for the *Gandharva* form.
101	4.1.1–5	This presumes a polygamous society. The role of one of several wives will be discussed in the next chapter. For Gonardiya see 1.1.11–12. The wife giving due regard to the husband's sisters is an orthodox social expectation to this day.
103	4.1.31–35	J explains that the chaff can be used for polishing things, broken grain for feeding pet birds, gruel for the servants and charcoal for firing iron pots.
105	4.2.1–2	Similar and variant conditions in which a man may take another wife are also mentioned in M (9.80–81) and legal texts like *Yajnavalkya Smriti* (1.73).
107–8	4.2.31	The Sanskrit word, here translated as 'the remarried woman', is *punarbhu*. She is described in M (9.175) as a remarried

NOTES

woman who was abandoned by her previous husband or separated from him of her own will. Manu's recent translator (see Introduction), Patrick Olivelle, points out that the broader term is *parapurva*, a woman who has previously had sexual relations with a man. But this term has a sevenfold classification, only three of which are called *punarbhu*. The others refer to wanton or unchaste women. M also specifies the inheritance rights of a *punarbhu*'s children, thus recognizing her status.

110	4.2.62	According to J the wives live in the central part of the harem, with the remarried women, the courtesans and the dancing girls living in successively outer parts.
115	5.1.1–2	Earlier discussed in 1.5.4–27.
116	5.1.8–12	For Gonikaputra see Note on V's Predecessors.
116–17	5.1.17–42	For the doe and the elephant women and their sexual impulses, see 2.1.1–7. The last sentence shows concern for Dharma while pursuing Kama, as does 'right' and 'wrong' in 5.1.8–12.
117	5.1.43–49	J glosses the aforesaid elements as follows. Related to nobility: love for husband, concern for children, onset of age and concern for Dharma. To inability: sympathy, self-disgust, absence of opportunity. To respect: shyness, comradeship, doubt. To lack of respect: suspicion, revulsion, contempt, scorn. To the man's disrespect: anger, alarm, his care for friends. To fear: diffidence, the doe woman's

apprehension, the elephant woman's concern, fear of the family.

119	5.1.55	This could be a general statement or refer in particular to the woman's desire.
122	5.2.19–22	The methods with a virgin girl are described in 3.3.6–8.
126–7	5.4.2–8	For the doe woman and the others see 2.1.1–4.
127	5.4.9–12	See note to 5.1.8–12 for Gonikaputra. V's own opinion about using a messenger is at 5.2.1–3.
127	5.4.13–15	Ahalya, the wife of a sage, was seduced by Indra, the king of the gods. The story occurs in the epic *Ramayana*. For Shakuntala, see note to 3.5.1–2. Avimaraka's love affair with a princess is the subject of a play with the same name by the celebrated *c.* second-century CE Sanskrit dramatist Bhasa. For the sixty-four arts see note to 1.3.13–16.
128	5.4.32–35	See Note on V's Predecessors for these persons cited by V. Auddalaki is the patronymic of Shvetaketu.
128–9	5.4.36–41	The supplication, as explained by J, is the imprint on the cloth of the man's palms which he would otherwise join together to beseech the woman.
129	5.4.42–44	'Times of trouble' are notably not excluded from the list of occasions for a romantic rendezvous. As to the venue, V is both prudent and cynical.
130–31	5.4.54–60	The seduction of a woman's lover by her

own scheming messenger is a common subject in Sanskrit erotic poetry. Good examples are available at vv. 203–207 of the translation of the fifteenth-century verse anthology *Subhashitavali*, published by Penguin Books India (2007).

131–2	5.4.64–66	The 'other person' is the one who has sent the go-between to the woman he desires. In the next verse he is mentioned as 'the man'.
133	5.5.5–10	The spinning-master supervised poor women who made their livings by spinning yarn.
135–6	5.5.28–35	See Note on Place Names.
136	5.5.36–37	The six inner enemies are lust, anger, greed, arrogance, infatuation and envy. They are often enumerated in Sanskrit verses, for example in the *c.* sixth-century *Kiratarjuniya* (1.9) of the celebrated poet Bharavi.
136–7	5.6.1–5	The Sanskrit word *apadravya*, literally a bad thing, is translated here as dildo. It is glossed in J 6.6.4 as an artificial device tied to the hips.
139–40	5.6.29–38	See Note on Place Names.
141	5.6.46–48	In effect, the descriptions here are not to be viewed as recommendations. Also see 7.2.54–55.
145–6	6.1.7–9	The professional companions, jesters and hangers-on or parasites included in this list of a woman's helpers were earlier described in 1.4.31–35 as the helpers of a man.
147	6.1.15–16	The first sentence refers to the qualities of both women and men given at 6.1.10–14.

But the passage as a whole refers only to men. The word *vayasasya*, here translated as 'breath which smells of crows,' literally means 'crow-mouth' and could refer to the bird's indiscriminate eating habits.

150   6.2.3–11   Leftover flowers could be those from the last encounter or from a ceremony of worship.

150–51   6.2.12–19   For the sixty-four arts see 2.2.1–5 and 2.10.34–39.

151   6.2.27–32   Like saying 'God bless you' when someone sneezes.

152–3   6.2.53–61   The first sentence expresses the wish that they be together again in her next life.

153   6.2.62–71   The crows are fed on the occasion for good luck.

153–4   6.2.72–76   For Dattaka see Note on V's Predecessors.

155   6.3.14–20   The last sentence, according to J, amplifies a quotation the commentary cites from Dattaka, cf. note above.

159   6.4.14–16   The penultimate sentence puns on the word *raga* which has the meanings of both passion and colour.

167–8   6.6.5–12   This is set in the context of the three ends of human life mentioned at 1.1.1–5 and 1.2.1–13.

168–9   6.6.17–20   Commenting on 6.6.20, J calculates twenty-four combined consequences.

170–71   6.6.34–40   For Auddalaki and Babhravya see Note on V's Predecessors.

172   6.6.50–51   Compare with 6.5.28–32, where courtesans

are placed in three grades on the basis of their profits.

175–6 7.1.8–11   *Atharva Veda* is the fourth of the four *Vedas* which are regarded by the faithful as *shruti* or revealed scripture. Its verses also include incantations for magical and prescriptions for medicinal use.

180   7.1.49–51   The *Veda* mentioned here is glossed by J as *Atharva Veda*, for which see the preceding note. *Ayurveda* is a separate later text on health and longevity.

180–81 7.2.1–3   For intense and dull sexual impulses see 2.1.5–7.

181   7.2.4–13   Another artificial device is mentioned at 5.6.1–5 for use between women, and translated as dildo. Here the device appears to be one or more rings, a beaded string or a sheath in which the penis is enclosed.

181–2 7.2.14–24   The suggestion here is for the insertion of variously shaped objects into a cut made on the penis. From J's gloss to 7.2.16 it would appear that the cut is made after pushing back the foreskin.

183   7.2.32–34   Methods presumably for getting rid of an unwanted lover. See 6.3.42.

183–4 7.2.35–42   The phrase 'turns it black again' has been used following J's gloss of the words in 7.2.39 which mean literally, 'restoration of the hair'.

185–6 7.2.54–55   This is a general disclaimer, as also in 5.6.46–48.

Note on Vatsyayana's Predecessors

Vatsyayana takes care to mention earlier authorities. The list in the *Kama Sutra* (1.1.8–12) begins with Nandi, the mythical servant of the great god Shiva. The nine names which follow his are of more mundane figures, probably with some historical basis as in several cases they are also mentioned in other works. These are the teachers Shvetaketu, Babhravya, Dattaka, Charayana, Suvarnanabha, Ghotakamukha, Gonardiya, Gonikaputra and Kuchumara.

Shvetaketu is a Vedic sage. He features in a number of episodes in the literature of the *Upanishads*, composed from *c.* sixth century BCE or earlier, though the dating is still uncertain. The best-known story is in the *Chhandogya Upanishad* (6.12.1–3 and 6.13.1–3). In it he is the earnest young son of the hermit Uddalaka Aruni, who explains to him the unity of all existence (*tat tvam asi* or 'that thou art') with dramatic examples of the seed of a tree and salt dissolved in water.

In the *Brihadaranyaka Upanishad* (6.2.13) Shvetaketu is mentioned incidentally as sending his father to a king, who compares offerings in the sacred fire with sexual intercourse. In the later epic *Mahabharata* (1.113.9–20) he is depicted as a sage involved in originating the institution of marriage in a promiscuous society, having seen his own mother led away by a man other than his father. In the *Kama Sutra* his views are cited on various subjects: on female orgasm (2.1.10–15); on the go-between's role (5.4.32); and on calculating gains and losses (6.6.34–35). He is mostly mentioned with his patronymic Auddalaki.

Babhravya is the only teacher identified in the *Kama Sutra* with a place, in this instance Panchala, the old name for the land between the Rivers Ganga and Yamuna in the north Indian plains. While he is cited only once (2.10.34–39), the *Kama Sutra*'s text has numerous references to his followers (1.5.30, 2.1.18, 2.2.4–5, 2.2.21–22, 2.6.19–22, 5.4.32–35, 5.4.42–44, 5.6.43–45, 6.3.36–40, 7.2.4–7). It would appear that he founded a school and remained well known in succeeding centuries. His own work is quoted by Yashodhara, the thirteenth-century CE commentator on the *Kama Sutra* (5.6.42); and the fourteenth-century work on erotics, *Panchasayaka*, mentions him as an authority on the subject.

Commenting on the *Kama Sutra* (6.3.20), Yashodhara also quotes from the work of Dattaka, who is further mentioned as an authority in the *Kuttanimatam* (vv. 77 and 123), the eighth-century account of courtesans written in Kashmir. A legend has him adopted as a child by a courtesan, and Vatsyayana says that he wrote his work at the behest of the courtesans of Pataliputra. He cites Dattaka on lovers' quarrels (2.10.51) and on methods of dispensing with a lover (6.3.43–44).

Kama Sutra cites Charayana (1.4.7–8, 1.5.22–27) on a gentleman's life and on permissible women. Suvarnanabha is cited (1.5.22–27, 2.4.4–6, 2.5.34–35, 2.6.23–35, 2.8.14–16) mainly on sexual union. Charayana is also named in the fourth-century BCE *Artha Shastra*, together with the teacher Ghotakamukha. The latter is often cited in the *Kama Sutra* (1.5.22–27, 3.1.3, 3.1.8–13, 3.2.13–17, 3.3.3–5, 3.4.26–31), mainly on choosing a bride and the first night after marriage.

The names of Gonardiya and Gonikaputra are also found in the *c.* first-century BCE work on grammar, *Mahabhashya* of Patanjali. The former is cited in the *Kama Sutra* (1.5.22–27, 4.1.1–5, 4.2.28–30, 4.2.33–35), chiefly on the roles of wives. He is also quoted in the fourteenth-century commentary by Mallinatha on descriptions of debauchery in Kalidasa's poem *Raghuvamsha* (19.16 and 19.29). Gonikaputra is cited in the *Kama Sutra* on permissible and avoidable women (1.5.4–7, 1.5.30–31), on wives of other men (5.1.8–12, 5.4.9–12, 5.4.42–44) and on guarding the harem (5.6.39–42). He is also mentioned as an authority in the twelfth-century work on erotics *Rat-*

irahasya (2.1–17). There are no specific citations for Kuchumara, who is named as the author of a separate work on esoteric subjects.

It is thus clear that some of these personages are known both from works predating the *Kama Sutra* and from others which followed it. Some of their writings were also available in the following centuries. This points to their historicity, though little else is known about them.

Note on Place Names

In the course of its descriptions of regional characteristics and customs the *Kama Sutra* mentions people from different places (for example at 1.1.8–10, 2.3.4–6, 2.4.9–11, 2.5.21–33, 2.6.22, 2.9.27–32, 2.10.10–13, 5.5.28–29, 5.5.30–35 and 5.6.29–38). Some of these place names are still in use, though the areas or the inhabitants to which they refer may no longer be in the same location. The following identification is based mainly on information derived from the glosses on relevant *Kama Sutra* passages (indicated within brackets) in the commentary *Jayamangala* (J) and from the appendix on geographical names in Apte's Sanskrit–English Dictionary (Delhi, 1965). The names are given in alphabetical order.

Abhira J (2.5.21) identifies it with the land of Kurukshetra near modern Delhi. The area is placed in the Vindhya Hills in central India, too. The name is also used for a people or tribe mainly of dairy farmers.

Ahichhatra A city possibly in the area of Kurukshetra.

Andhra A region south of the Vindhya Hills, now the name of a state in southern India and its people.

Anga Identified with present north Bihar. J (5.6.37) places it to the east of the River Mahanadi.

Aparanta The coastal land between the Western Ghat hills and the Arabian Sea.

Avanti The area north of the River Narmada in present western

Madhya Pradesh. Its capital was Ujjayini at the site of modern Ujjain.

Bahlika Identified with the region of Balkh in northern Afghanistan or with people from there.

Dravida Placed by J (2.5.31) to the south of Karnataka. This would correspond to present Tamilnadu. The name is still in use in cultural terms.

Gauda Present northern Bengal.

Kalinga The southern part of the present state of Orissa in eastern India.

Kashi An ancient city on the River Ganga in the present state of Uttar Pradesh, on the site of modern Varanasi. The name is still in use.

Kosala Corresponds to the eastern part of present Uttar Pradesh.

Kotta J (5.5.29) names it as a place in the present state of Gujarat.

Lata An area to the west of the River Narmada in present Gujarat.

Madhya Desha Literally, the central region. Described in J (2.5.21) as the land between the Himalayas and the Vindhyas. Corresponds to the bulk of the Gangetic plain in north India.

Maharashtra A part of the present state of this name in west and central India. J (2.5.29) places it between the River Narmada and the land of Karnataka.

Malava The region of present Malwa in central India adjacent to Avanti.

Panchala Identified with the land between the Rivers Ganga and Yamuna in north India.

Saketa A city in Kosala. J (2.9.30) identifies it with Ayodhya, a name still current.

Saurashtra The region of the same name in present Gujarat.

Sindhu The region of Sindh in southern Pakistan.

Stri Rajya Literally, the kingdom of women. Refers perhaps to an area with a matriarchal society in a location still to be identified.

Surasena J (2.9.32) places it to the south of Kaushambi, a city which existed close to present Allahabad in Uttar Pradesh. It has also been placed in the western part of the same state in the area around present Mathura.

Vanavasa   Literally, a forest habitation. Placed by J (2.5.32) to the east of the Konkan region of present Maharashtra.

Vanga   Present eastern Bengal.

Vatsagulma   It has been suggested (A.K. Warder, *Indian Kavya Literature*, vol.3, Delhi, 1990, 1265) that this was the capital of Vidarbha during the *c.* fourth-century Vakataka empire, but the location remains unidentified.

Vidarbha   An area between the Rivers Krishna and Narmada corresponding to the region of Berar. The name is still in use.

The *Kama Sutra* also mentions (2.5.30 and 2.9.31) women and men of *nagara*, that is 'The City'. This is identified in J with Pataliputra, which was long an imperial capital in ancient India, situated near present Patna in the state of Bihar. Vatsyayana's references to the people and the practices of 'the south' and 'the east' most probably indicate areas in these directions beyond the Madhya Desha.

Select Bibliography

Sanskrit

Kamasutra of Vatsyayana, with the commentary Jayamangala of Yashodhara
— ed. Pandit Durgaprasada (Nirnaya Sagar Press, Bombay, 1891)
— ed. Damodar Goswami Shastri (Kashi Sanskrit Series, Benaras, 1912)
— ed. With Hindi commentary by Devdatta Shastri (Chaukhamba Sanskrit Sansthan, Varanasi, 1964)
— ed. With the *Purusharthaprabha* Hindi commentary by Madhavacharya (Khemraj Shrikrishnadas, Mumbai, 1995)
Kamasutra of Vatsyayana, ed. with English translation and notes by Radhavallabha Tripathi (Pratibha Prakashan, Delhi, 2005)

English Translations

The Kama Sutra of Vatsyayana, tr. Sir Richard Burton.
— printed for Hindoo Kama Shastra Society (London and Benaras, 1883)
— With Foreword by Santha Rama Rau and Introduction by J. W. Spellman (E.P. Dutton & Co., New York, 1962)
— ed. John Muirhead-Gould, Introduction by Don Moraes (Panther Books, London, 1963)

— ed. with Preface by W.G. Archer, Introduction by K.M. Panikkar (Berkeley Books, New York, 1966)

Kama-sutra of Vatsyayana: the Hindu Art of Love, tr. B.M. Basu, rev. S.L. Ghosh (Medical Book Co., Calcutta, 1959)

Kamasutra, tr. S.C. Upadhyaya, Foreword by Moti Chandra (D.B. Taraporevala & Sons, Bombay, 1963)

Kama Sutra, ed. Mulk Raj Anand and Lance Dane (Sanskrit Pratishthan for Arnold Heinemann, Delhi, 1982)

The Complete Kama Sutra, tr. into French by Alain Danielou and by him into English with the help of Kenneth Harry (Park Street Press, Rochester, Vt, 1994)

Kamasutra, tr. Wendy Doniger and Sudhir Kakar (Oxford University Press, New York, 2002)

Kamasutra of Vatsyayana, ed. and tr. Radhavallabha Tripathi (Pratibha Prakashan, Delhi, 2005)

Other Reading

Auboyer, Jeanine, *Daily Life in Ancient India* (Phoenix Press, London, 2002)

Basham, A.L., *The Wonder that was India* (Grove Press, New York, 1954)

Bhattacharyya, Narendra Nath, *History of Indian Erotic Literature* (Munshiram Manoharlal, New Delhi, 1975)

Chakladar, Haran Chandra, *Social Life in Ancient India: Studies in Vatsyayana's Kamasutra* (Sushil Gupta, Calcutta, 1929)

De, Sushil Kumar, *Ancient Indian Erotics and Erotic Literature* (Firma K.L. Mukhopadhyaya, Calcutta, 1959)

Hampiholi, Viswanath K., *Kamashastra in Classical Sanskrit Literature* (Ajanta Publications, Delhi, 1988)

Keith, A.B., *History of Sanskrit Literature* (Oxford University Press, Oxford, 1928)

McConnachie, James, *The Book of Love – The Story of the Kamasutra* (Metropolitan Books, New York, 2008)

Meyer, J.J., *Sexual Life in Ancient India* (Barnes and Noble, New York, 1953)

Olivelle, Patrick, ed. and tr., *Manu's Code of Law* (Oxford University Press, New York, 2005)

Pannikar, K.M., *Studies in Indian History* (Asia Publishing House, Bombay, 1963)

Rangarajan, L.N., ed. and tr., *The Artha Shastra of Kautilya* (Penguin Books India, New Delhi, 1994)

Warder, A.K., *Indian Kavya Literature*, vol. 1 (Motilal Banarsidass, Delhi, 1974)

Winternitz, Maurice, tr. Subhadra Jha, *History of Indian Literature*, vol. 3 (Motilal Banarsidass, Delhi, 1967)